YOGA: WHAT IT IS AND [WHAT] MAKES IT USEFUL TO [YOU]

YOGA, MEDICINE AND P[...]

HOW YOU CAN BENEFIT [IN MANY] WAYS FROM DAILY USE O[F YOGA] TECHNIQUES

YOGA AND SEX

YOGA AND A LONG LIFE

'This is a straightforward account of the benefits to be derived from the practice of Yoga. Mr. Dunne sticks to essentials'
Oxford Mail

'Yoga is a technique of mental and physical disciplines that may readily be incorporated into everybody's day-to-day existence. It can be practised at any age'
The Psychologist

Desmond Dunne
Principal, The Insight School of Yoga

Yoga Made Easy

MAYFLOWER
GRANADA PUBLISHING
London Toronto Sydney New York

Published by Granada Publishing Limited
in Mayflower Books 1971
Reprinted 1973 (twice), 1974, 1976, 1978

ISBN 0 583 19735 3

First published in Great Britain by
Souvenir Press Ltd 1962
Copyright © Prentice-Hall Incorporated 1961

Granada Publishing Limited
Frogmore, St Albans, Herts AL2 2NF
and
3 Upper James Street, London W1R 4BP
1221 Avenue of the Americas, New York, NY10020, USA
117 York Street, Sydney, NSW 2000, Australia
100 Skyway Avenue, Toronto, Ontario, Canada M9W 3A6
Trio City, Coventy Street, Johannesburg 2001, South Africa
CML Centre, Queen & Wyndham, Auckland 1, New Zealand

Made and printed in Great Britain by
Hunt Barnard Printing Ltd
Aylesbury, Bucks
Set in Monotype Plantin

Contents

Illustrations

What Yoga Can Do for You

Yoga is an ancient health-art developed and perfected over the centuries by the Sages and Wise Men of ancient India. Yoga is *not* a religion, a metaphysical doctrine, or a philosophy. It is not magic or mysticism, although the amazing improvements it can make in your health, your appearance and your youthfulness may often seem magical, even miraculous.

For thousands of years the Yogis of India have used the simple, reasonable principles of Yoga to regain the zest and enthusiasm and good health of their youth, to preserve into middle age the clear-thinking and sound physique of manhood, and to continue enjoying *even in old age* the resilience, healthfulness, and well-being of their younger years.

Yoga can take years off your face and years from your body— and add years to your life. There are certain secret methods by which the Yogis keep the flexibility and "spring" of early youth in their joints and muscles and limbs well into the declining years. It is a common sight to see, in the crowded, colorful streets of Bombay or New Delhi, Yogis well into their seventies and even their eighties, with the straight, graceful posture of a boy, walking with the elastic, springy step of youth . . . with firm, healthy bodies, their hair dark and glossy and unstreaked with grey. Firm, unlined faces . . . clear, undimmed eyes.

Not only does Yoga make you look and feel years younger, years healthier, but it lends your body superb healthiness. This system of Yoga does not demand difficult positions and postures, uncomfortable exercises or strenuous diets. This is where it differs from every other book on Yoga previously published. It describes the simple, easy, "common-sense" secrets of *using the natural health God gave you*. It works like magic because it enables the body to realize its full potential of good health.

You know that Nature built into your body certain natural safeguards against disease, certain "defense mechanisms" for self-repair. Well, modern Yoga helps the body's machinery function smoothly, efficiently, at peak performance. It encourages your body to derive every last possible atom of nutritive value from the food you now eat (so different from the natural diet of your ancestors) ... to get every second of refreshment and rest from your sleep . . . to attain regularity, relief from little aches and pains, the ability to sleep deep and wake refreshed that can make the difference from feeling "pretty good" to feeling "terrific!"

Yoga assists *all* your muscles and bones and organs to operate at top masculine or female vigor. Yoga stimulates into peak performance the latent abilities of your body to throw off the attacks of disease, the psychosomatic "nervous illnesses" that nag and plague millions. Do you suffer from insomnia, "nerves"? Are you without appetite? Do you find it hard to relax? Do you smoke too much, feel "worn out" by afternoon, find as you grow older that you cannot enjoy full life and day to day vitality? Yoga has the amazing power to refresh and relax you, soothe your nerves, calm your mind, give you the serenity and strength and inner stamina that is part of the "Magic of the East."

Yoga prevents the premature grey in your hair, the ugly wrinkles in your face. It tightens those sagging muscles that give you that "tired look." It puts new zest in your appetite, brings back the sparkle in your eyes—gives that wonderful sensation of feeling "fit as a fiddle."

For far too long the secret wisdom and lore of this ancient art has been denied to men and women of the Western world. I have devoted years of study and experiment to the cause of *revising and simplifying* the ancient practices of Yoga and to making them accessible to modern Americans. I have *adapted, modified* and "*streamlined*" Yoga so that it will be of *the very highest possible value to you today*. In so doing, I have taken full cognizance of modern advances in nutrition, vitamin-therapy, health foods, and the new systems of diet and exercise, as well as the most recent medical knowledge and research into methods of revitalizing the human body and halting the "aging process."

You want a full life. You want to feel well. You want energy, vitality, staying power. All these can be yours. This system of Yoga applies age-old secrets to everyday life at the modern tempo. It tells how only a few minutes' easy, practical application can restore your lost youth . . . put new zest into your undertakings . . . and enable you to enjoy to the full a sense of health, energy and creative living which will make all the difference to your future happiness.

Desmond Dunne

PART I

THE THEORY OF YOGA

What It Is
And What Makes It
Useful to Everyone

CHAPTER I

Why Yoga?

As recently as a century ago, when the average life expectancy throughout the Western world was less than forty years, people gave little thought to keeping fit. Life was simply not long enough. The few men and women who lived into their eighties and nineties were thought old souls of whom it was said that they were so mean nothing would kill them.

Today the picture has changed. On the one hand, science and medicine have combined to lessen the hazards to which we are exposed. Plagues have been wiped out. Anti-biotics and other miracle drugs are conquering diseases long considered incurable. Surgery is capable of life-saving magic. Our life expectancy has very nearly doubled and continues to rise.

On the other hand, we have acquired an entirely new set of problems. Even as the years of our lives stretch out longer, existence becomes infinitely more complex. By its very nature, twentieth century civilization makes this inevitable. The Atomic Age is hardly a relaxed age. We circle the globe in a matter of hours, we talk of trips to the moon as the reality of tomorrow—but we also know that tomorrow's wars, unless prevented, will be on a scale to wipe out continents.

On the personal level, our urban civilization brings with it tensions virtually unknown in our grandparents' time. We tend to live on the run, geared to split-second timing, to noise, to newscasts every hour on the hour, to phones jangling and cars honking, subway trains, deadlines and keeping up with the Joneses and seldom sufficient rest, relaxation or sleep. None of this is conducive to peace of mind. As for our physical conditions, as fast as the human body is enabled, through technical advances, to last longer, it falls prey to a new, totally different roster of ills.

Look around you and compare the medical picture with what it once was: Smallpox has all but vanished, tuberculosis is rapidly being wiped out, pneumonia rarely kills, death in childbirth is no longer something to fear. But now it is the diseases of old age and of tension that are the evening. Today heart trouble is the number one killer. Ulcers, arthritis, allergies, and allergic respiratory disturbances—not to mention mental illness of every variety—plague the young, the not-so-young and the elderly.

But since the world we live in is the only world we have, and since we cannot individually do much to change it, the next best thing is to learn to adjust to it with some degree of comfort. True, we cannot very well go bucolic, escape to some Thoreauvian Walden, some Shangri-La of our own making. Nor can we shut our eyes, close our ears, turn off our emotions enabling us to remain impervious to the life around us. We probably wouldn't want to do that even if we could, for who but a born hater would deliberately choose indifference to those very qualities which make us warm human beings?

Fortunately there does exist an answer to this problem. It is possible for anyone who will only take the trouble to learn to live serenely in our Age of Anxiety. Within easy reach is a key to living out one's allotted span of three-score-and-ten or more, enjoying all the while a vigorous mind in a vigorous body, both of them functioning to the very limit of their potential. The key to such well-being is Yoga.

Yoga, you say? But that's some kind of Eastern magic, or maybe a religion! Yoga is a Hindu with an exotic headdress, climbing a rope firmly anchored in mid-air. It's a man walking barefoot over hot coals or lying on a bed of nails.

Nothing of the sort! The misconceptions about Yoga are many, and naturally what sticks in the minds of most people is the flamboyant, or what we might call the circus approach. But this we can happily leave to the tricksters. The truth has nothing whatever in common with any spectacular nonsense. True

Yoga philosophy and Yoga health practices are sane, serious, utilitarian and easily applicable to our own daily lives.

As far back as the days of Marco Polo travelers in the East returned home with tales of men they had met totally unlike ordinary mortals. These were sages and philosophers, described as being singularly serene, detached, apparently unaffected by the ordinary stresses and strains of living, indifferent to pain and frequently possessed of certain extraordinary sensory powers. Their concentration, their physical control, their insight were amazing. Their hands could heal, their spirit travel to distant places. And while they lived to be unbelievably old, they seldom looked their age. Invariably they were held in the highest esteem.

The sages whom the travelers described were Hindu *Yogis* —a *Yogi* being a follower of *Yoga*, the ancient school of philosophy whose founder, Pantanjali, lived in the third century B.C. Often these men were also *Gurus*, or teachers, each of whom had dedicated a lifetime to the kind of study and practice which made him an outstanding figure in his chosen way of life. The claims made for them, fantastic as these may sound, need not necessarily have been exaggerated. In fact the *modern* traveler in India will still come upon their counterparts, for such men do exist, as even the most skeptical of scientists will not deny. Nor are they magicians, even though to the uninitiated they may *seem* to have attained truly supernatural powers.

In a later chapter we shall briefly come back to them— discuss, analyze and attempt to explain some of their more striking achievements—but only in order to give the student a general idea of what the profound study of Yoga does make possible by way of ultimate goals. Right now let us make it very clear, however, that no one advocates setting up such goals for the Occidental student. This is not the purpose of our book. Indeed nobody could hope to achieve or even approximate them without devoting a lifetime to their single-minded pursuit. Certainly it could never be done without a *Guru* for a guide.

For the average Westerner there exists an altogether different approach—a serviceable adaptation, as distillation of Eastern methods, which for purposes of clarity I have chosen to call *Yogism*. Stripped to bedrock, here is a technique in the form of mental and physical disciplines that may readily be incorporated into our day-by-day existence. One needn't make a career of it. Thus Yogism may and does serve as an easy, pleasant road to self-discovery and well-being and will help anyone willing to approach it with an open mind. Yet there is no need to devote more time to it each day than it takes to smoke a cigarette, drink a second cup of coffee and listen to newscasts after breakfast, lunch and dinner.

If you are an average man or woman coping with just average problems, here is what you are doubtless up against: Your day is too short. You rush to work in the morning and home at night, fighting your way through crowds and traffic tangles. You work under pressure on the job or in the home, and at the end of the day you are up against more pressures: Bills must be paid, expenses budgeted, chores taken care of after hours; your children bring their problems to you; the house-hold absorbs all your energy; family life makes endless demands on your emotional and physical resources. And even though you love your kin and give of yourself willingly, there are times when things simply pile up and threaten to overwhelm you.

The same holds true for your work-world: In the course of any single day you are up against a dozen unforeseen complications—there are delays, disappointments, errors, misunderstandings, irritations and similar minor crises. Heaven help you if, on top of all this, a major crisis looms. All at once you feel driven beyond your capacity.

Different people have different ways of responding to all these pressures. Some panic, others lose their temper or become paralyzed. The physiological reactions vary too, but chances are they will manifest themselves (in addition to snapping at others or indulging in what the French call a *crise de nerfs*, freely translated as the "screaming meemies") in symptoms such as headache, insomnia, backaches, nervous ticks, hives, stomach upsets. Keep the tensions up, let them begin to feel insoluble, and the body protests by escaping into psychogenic illnesses—illnesses that are very real indeed, but whose causes are mental rather than strictly physical. Next come the perpetual frowns, the wrinkles, the greying hair, a general sense of defeat and of growing old before one's time.

Yet none of this misery is inevitable, if you only make up your mind not to let it get its insidious hold on you. That's where the practice of Yoga can be of such enormous help. Think of Yoga as a tool that will help you banish fear, and the fear of fear. Think of it as a key to spiritual freedom. Give yourself a chance to reshape your own destiny.

At first it may sound far-fetched to claim that taking up the practice of Yogism or any other *ism* might help solve or even hold out the promise of solutions to objective problems. What, you may well ask, can a few breathing exercises, a few posture routines, bring to bear on whether or not the family budget can be stretched to cover the cost of those braces the dentist just said Johnny needs at once, without cutting into his precious college fund? And will it help build the addition to the house without which it will simply be murder to let your mother-in-law come to live with you?

Of course no one suggests such over-simplification. But consider this: Inasmuch as body and mind—or, if you will, the purely physical and the purely mental processes—are part of a single organic whole, it stands to reason that whatever affects the one will of necessity, directly or indirectly, affect the other. Therefore, just as emotional tensions often result in physical illness, so a state of physical well-being and relaxation can result in a more reasoned, relaxed approach to one's emotional problems and the tensions they bring on. And that, of course, is the first important step to being able to deal with them—the first step out of your quandary and in the direction of a solution.

But a more relaxed outlook on life is only one of the benefits that Yoga has to offer. *To follow its precepts means learning to get more out of yourself, in every respect.* For instance, proper breathing and relaxation, the very cornerstone of all Yoga teachings, result in deeper, more beneficial sleep and a general sense of restfulness and well-being; and these in turn enable one to function at the very optimum of one's abilities. It is not just a question of building greater resistance to emotional storms with their possible aftermath of psychogenic illness; a rested mind and a rested body are, as any doctor will tell you, the best kind of health insurance. So starts an entire beneficial cycle: a healthy body means a better-functioning body, it means added tone, improved functioning of the glands; and that in turn means better metabolism, muscle tone, skin tone, elimination and general vitality and vigor. It means eyes that sparkle, hair that shines and 'appetites time will not dull. In fact, it means slowing up the entire process of deterioration which we call aging and which in Western man starts so pitifully early.

As for the spiritual and mental results of Yoga practice, these soon become manifest in a fresh ability to make the most of one's inner resources. As one's powers of relaxation increase, there follows an enormous improvement in concentration. Soon the student finds himself in control of his thoughts instead of being controlled by them. And so instead of living at about ten percent of capacity, as do most people, he learns to live at one hundred percent, fully, deeply. He begins to do away with the fragmentation of his emotional wherewithal, escaping the whip of self-drive which can be so destructive, learning instead to think and feel clearly so that he wastes no more precious time in letting his mind wander in circles. Rather, he makes friends with himself until his whole organism functions as an integrated, positive whole, not a house divided. In psychoanalytical language so popular today, one might say it all adds up to the conquest of what has come to be recognized as the "neurotic personality of our times."

We can also put it another way:

Through the centuries our ancestors spent years of their time and energy, and sometimes large fortunes, looking for the elixir of youth—only their search for the secret of how to make gold out of baser metals was ever pursued with as much passion. Men were willing to sell their souls to the devil for it, women to bargain away their chastity; expeditions traveled to the four corners of the earth searching for it, hoping for magic wells and magic spells and poultices. The prize, if found, was to be a promise of physical perfection without end: beauty that did not fade, an ever-supple, lovely body, a face without lines. For the man it meant undiminished vitality and sexual powers; for the woman the allure of a Helen of Troy. Or, translated into everyman's ultimate desire, it added up to never-ending zest for life, a boundless joy.

Well, the men who searched for magic formulae were doomed to failure. It was the Yoga sages who, without any magic whatsoever, offered the world something of this secret. For in reality it isn't *eternal* life that man longs for, but rather a long, good, useful life lived to the full and without fear— fear of pain, of dependence, of invalidism and weakness and all the other miseries which can make old age a burden and an indignity. It is a life so organized and so satisfying that in its twilight a person will be content to let go without regrets and without a sense of leaving too much undone. This, in many ways, is or can be our ultimate achievement.

Such goals, based on the principle of a perfect marriage between a mind at peace and a body that remains sound and active long after middle-age and old age would normally have begun to make their inroads, are not unrealistic for the student of Yoga. Once you learn to live without tensions, you discover your own optimum potential and are on the way, though without urgency, to live up to it; in short, once you begin to achieve that inner harmony which will allow you to stop living at odds with yourself, you will find your entire viewpoint changing. Your relationships with others will grow more harmonious and satisfying too, for nothing is so attractive to people as a harmonious personality. Naturally the world around you will then become a more attractive place for you to live in.

People often ask, understandably enough, whether there aren't some limitations as to the time of life when the study of Yoga may begin. Fortunately, the answer to this question is an emphatic NO. You can begin at any age. Old people may take it up as well as the young, and even children have benefited by it.

There are bound to be differences in approach, yet there is nothing rigid nor schematic about the study of Yoga itself, and certainly *Yogism*, that modified form adapted specially to our Occidental tempo, can be further varied to meet the needs of every individual. True, when it comes to certain advanced exercises and postures, an octogenarian will not be likely to try tying himself up in knots like a limber eighteen-year old. But just for the record let me mention a lady of seventy-four, and another who is eighty, both of whom make it a practice to do the headstand for a few minutes each day. Both are fairly recent students—which ought to prove a point. On the other hand the very young, who with their wonderfully elastic limbs and limber joints are often able to approach the most difficult Yoga postures in the spirit of play, will gain little from such practices if permitted to perform them like acrobatic stunts. For, the prime purpose of Yoga is a re-education of one's mental processes along with the physical. Therefore, encouraging children to participate will only serve a purpose if it will teach them the habit of relaxing, help them grow up relaxed. Considering a child's apparently inexhaustible supply of self-perpetuating energy, this is not easy; but neither is it impossible provided the teaching is by example and emulation. Relax with them, and they will absorb the essence of what you are trying to get across. Above all, always keep in mind that success is a relative matter—a matter of degree.

The Eastern Yogis claim that the best time of life to begin *Abbyasa*, or spiritual practice, is between the ages of twenty and forty. But this is only true of the student who means to dedicate his life to it. Since such undivided dedication is not our concern—since all we are after is a practical way to improve our day-by-day living—we can proceed at our own pace. Once this is completely clear, Yogism, or the adapted study of Yoga, can be integrated into anyone's scheme of things, beginning today, NOW.

CHAPTER II

What Yoga Is

By now the reader may have decided he has been promised the millennium. It might therefore be best before continuing with any further discussion to go back, examine Yoga in its varying forms and establish a common vocabulary in regard to it. We then can be completely clear on what this philosophy really is *and what it is not*—also on what it bases its claims and which of its teachings are applicable and useful to us.

Let us begin with a working definition: *Yoga is a method by which to obtain control of one's latent powers.* It offers the means to reach complete Self-realization. This the Yogis achieve by turning their thoughts inward, away from the objective world. The literal meaning of the Sanskrit word *Yoga* is *yoke.* Its earliest definition—a means for uniting the individual spirit with the Universal Spirit, or God if you will—may at first glance seem a contradiction of the other; but the confusion disappears once we take into account that realization of Self cannot be achieved without the recognition and acceptance of one's place in and relationship to the universe as a whole.

Yoga is very definitely *not* a religion: some Yogis are deeply religious, others are not. Many of its aspects are profoundly mystical, as is inevitable with any form of spiritual contemplation. But how the Yogi interprets his beliefs is an entirely personal matter. There are Brahmins among the Yogis, there are Christians, and there are Moslems, to name only a few. There are also philosophically-oriented persons with no formal religion.

The schools of Yoga are numerous, and even in the East

each student is generally attracted to that particular form of it which best answers his own particular needs. In many ways, too, the differences are largely a matter of emphasis for, as you will see, the various schools overlap to some extent. As you read on you will quickly be able to understand just why, as we have already pointed out, none is really suited unaltered to our Western temperament and the exigencies of our tempo of living.

A brief outline of the outstanding basic schools will illustrate this better than any flat statement of opinion.

First and most widespread, as well as the one best known in our hemisphere, is *Hatha Yoga*. The name, derived from the Sanskrit *Ha*, which stands for the female principle and *Tha*, the male principle, implies that this Yoga may be practiced by both men and women with the object of achieving complete control of the body. One feature of Hatha Yoga practice involves a number of such drastic, sometimes even painful, forms of spiritual and physical purification so impractical and alien to us that no attempt shall be made here to discuss them. For this purpose, the Western student need only be concerned with the kind of purification that may be attained by simple hygiene. This, like many other points which will be only briefly touched upon here, is something we shall return to in a subsequent chapter.

The second important feature of Hatha Yoga is the practice of *asanas* or postures. Again, since many asanas are difficult and require endless application and practice, there is little need to concern ourselves with all of them. Suffice it to mention that the basic ones number 84, a great many of them a total impossibility for most of us, be we young or old, athletically gifted or even double-jointed.

But the fact that we cannot hope to emulate the Hindu poses is of little import. The salient point here is that even a few of the simplest asanas, practiced daily together with a few *mudras* or contemplative poses, suffice to produce for us truly sensational results. You will readily understand the reason for this once you know the underlying principles for their practice.

In Part II we shall discuss the exercises in detail, illustrating with charts and photographs exactly how to do them correctly. But first a word about the difference between our own concept of exercise and that of the Yogis. To us exercise means exertion—the idea is to "work up a good sweat." Western athletic games aren't play, they are competition. And whether the competition is with others or with ourselves—how fast can I go, how far can I swim, how high can I climb this time?—inevitably the result is fatigue and strain along with the pleasure. In short, we make exercise hard work.

The Yogis have a concept almost diametrically opposed to ours. You will notice many of the asanas are named for animals: the lion, the fish, the tortoise, the peacock. This is because in devising them the Yogis based themselves on close observation of animal life. They borrowed from the animal world the secrets of alternate relaxing and tensing, something all living creatures save man seem to know how to do instinctively.

Watch a kitten at play: It wakes from a cat-nap, stretches, arches its back, yawns prodigiously, flicks its tail and instantly is chasing it. Whether or not it succeeds doesn't seem to matter. Next it will leap after a fly, change its mind, flop over and with the greatest nonchalance start washing a seemingly inaccessible spot in the middle of its back. Soon it is once more curled up in a ball or stretched out leggy and limp, one open eye proclaiming that it is not asleep—just relaxing.

The underlying emphasis in all asanas and mudras, then, is on relaxation—one might even say repose. And while at first glance it might seem that standing on one's head or sitting in the Lotus pose is anything but restful, this is only true of the initial stages of learning. Bear in mind that the body is always first slowly prepared for each pose and that the limbering-up process, which each student pursues at his own pace, is geared in such a way as not to overtax his capacities. By the time he is ready to practice an asana, certainly by the time he has mastered it, it really is relaxing as well as beneficial. Then the profound balance achieved by the body makes it possible for the mind to soar.

Yoga teaches that it is essential never to overdo, never to strain and tire. The motto here is always too little rather than too much—it is considered best to make haste slowly. The new student is invariably cautioned to proceed very gradually, for it is neither necessary nor desirable to establish records. He is also taught to rest between asanas and never to attempt anything beyond his capacities at the time.

Rhythmic deep breathing is an essential part of all exercises. Much more emphasis is put on breathing than is true of any of the Western schools of physical culture, since the Yogis understand that for purely physiological reasons deep breathing is a sure way to calm the nerves, and this in turn reduces tensions and improves concentration. One might say that the overall reason for combining deep breathing with asanas and mudras is that the Yogi, while purifying and disciplining his body, aims to bring his mind, too, under similar control.

Many Western students are content with the sheer physical well-being they are able to achieve, with no concern at all for the second aim, which is for mental and spiritual discipline. And indeed for many this may be all that is required. If you happen to be among those who have neither the time nor the temperament for further exploration, there is no reason to feel disturbed. Certainly under no circumstances is it necessary to adopt the everything-or-nothing attitude—no need to assume that unless you are willing to go further, the game isn't worth the candle.

As a matter of fact it would be extremely difficult, we should say impossible, to progress into the higher spiritual spheres of Yoga without the constant guidance of a *Guru*. In certain cases it would even be dangerous to try to go forward alone, and of this the Eastern student too is invariably warned. For the ultimate abstract psychic states reached in Yoga meditations are said to release forces as yet unknown to us, such as the Serpent Power or *Kundalini*, which we shall again discuss later. This power, released only when the subject is in a deep, trance-like state, is variously described as a vast sex power, as the source of creativity, even as the source of healing. Clearly it is no more a plaything for the neophyte or amateur than, for instance, hypnosis. Fortunately, the sensible adult will not be tempted to play such dangerous games. Our sole reason for mentioning these aspects of Yoga at this stage is to give the student some idea of the scope which even its most primary philosophies encompass.

Hatha Yoga, in common with other Yoga schools, teaches certain rules of conduct, or *yamas*. There are ten of these: *Ahimsa* or harmlessness, *Satya* or truthfulness, *Asteya* or non-stealing, *Bramacharya* or continence, *Kshama* or forbearance, *Dhriti* or fortitude, *Daya* or mercy, *Aarjvna* or straightfor-wardness, *Mithra* or moderation in diet, and *Suchi* or purity. There are also ten restrictions: *Tepas*, which means austerity, *Santosah*, cheerful bearing, *Shraddha*, faith, *Dana*, charitable disposition, *Satsanga*, good company, *Lajja*, modesty, *Mati*, sound mind, *Japa*, repetition of a divine name, *Ishwarachana*, worship of God, and *Vrata*, observance of vows.

From this it becomes self-evident that Hatha Yoga demands high personal standards. Overeating, unnecessary talk, im-pure associations, greed and delight alike must be eliminated. All this, obviously, is a good deal more austerity than we Oc-cidentals are generally ready to accept. Fortunately there is no need for extremes. As we have pointed out all along, this, like any other aspect of Yoga, for our immediate and practical use translates simply into an attitude of reasonable modera-tion. Of course, in time the advanced student may find him-self developing a certain attitude of indifference towards many of the demands of our competitive society—those demands which can so easily enslave the individual through emphasis on false values and later bring on discontent and a sense of failure if somewhat unrealistic, highly materialistic goals aren't achieved. If this does happen to you, you may well congratulate yourself. For, indifference to material success would be one of the many keys to that mental and emotional freedom without which well-being on any level may be considered inaccessible.

We have discussed Hatha Yoga at considerably greater

length and in more detail than other schools because this is the discipline we shall draw on in our practices. But the student will undoubtedly want to know a little about other Yogas, all of which place vastly more stress on non-physical disciplines. Thus *Japa Yoga* is a philosophy concerned exclusively with spiritual discipline; in one of its forms its practice consists of repeating a *Mantra*, or affirmation, over and over while dwelling deeply on its every significance. To accomplish this no mind-wandering at all is permissible, and since most persons' minds do wander to some extent the Japa Yogi, desirous of guarding against distraction, will often be found sitting motionless for hours on end, tailor fashion, while chanting the single whole syllable "Om." This chanting is done in conjunction with deep breathing, which admittedly does arrest mind-wandering so that the practitioner becomes drawn into himself in spiritual contemplation. But only the dedicated philosopher could be expected to pursue this practice. There is hardly a place for it in our Western world.

In Laya Yoga the student remains perfectly still, in a profound state of trance. Then, by means of the Kundalini power which at certain moments is released and joins with the Divine or ultimate power of the universe, he briefly achieves a state of perfect bliss. He must then quickly return to earth—to his normal state, if you will—otherwise he runs the danger of severing all connection with it. As we have already mentioned, this form of Yoga is not safe for anyone to practice who has not gained complete control over his emotions as well as over his mental processes.

Karma Yoga, another school that aims at final union with the Divine Source of All, advocates not the renouncement of all earthly work, but on the contrary its pursuit. It looks upon the body as "the good servant" of one's spiritual strivings. Essentially practical, Karma Yoga teaches helping others as a means of helping one's self. Karma being the principle of causality, this philosophy is essentially based on the law of Cause and Effect, on the recognition that for every action there is a corresponding reaction. In many ways it is not unlike early Christianity. As we sow, says Karma, so shall we reap.

Consequently, the tenets of Karma Yoga are a devotion of one's life to selfless service without any attachment whatever or consideration for rewards. The student of Karma is taught indifference to praise and blame alike. He may not accept gifts but must always work for work's own sake. His heart must be a garden filled with the flowers of good deeds. He must ever listen to the inner voice of his conscience for guidance, fear no one save the Divine power, and devote his life to his fellow-creatures. Mahatma Gandhi, who lived by such precepts, himself taught that there were no distinctions between menial and dignified work. He himself often performed the most menial tasks, and his was an example of the deepest humility, love and goodwill. While it is always unsatisfactory to suggest parallels, medieval anchorites and St. Francis of Assisi come to mind as we try to translate some of these attitudes into Western terms.

A further parallel is equally striking: Karma teaches that a man who lives a life of idleness and luxury cannot hope to help his fellows, for he is handicapped by enslavement to his *Indriyas* or sense powers. It follows that if he would become a true Karma Yogi he must cast outside his rich robes and take on the beggar's garb. This, after all, is not very different from the basic philosophy behind the words, "It is easier for a camel to pass through the needle's eye than for the rich man to enter the gates of heaven."

Still another school is *Jnana Yoga*, the Yoga of Knowledge as against that of Action. Jnana educates the mind to perceive Self and so free itself from all forms of delusion. It aims at the realization of the Supreme Self by means of learning to see the everyday world in its true proportions, making a complete cleavage between the objective manifestations of consciousness and the subjective working of the mind. Three thousand years after Hindu philosophers formulated this approach, modern Western psychiatry began to explore the same problems in the aboratory. The Yogis, however, attain their goal through purely

philosophical, meditative channels; they consider the first step
to be comprehension of what mind consists of, and the second
a mastery of all desire by the development of wisdom. Again,
such speculation is beyond the realm of ordinary people's
interests. Specifically, what Jnana says must follow is complete
non-attachment to the things of this world and constant
sacrifice of self to enlightenment. Jnana demands of the student
a technique of living so rigorous and an asceticism so extreme
as to be totally alien to most of us.

Bhakti Yoga is a system of intense devotion, with emphasis
on faith. The true follower of Bhakti is one who is free from
both guilt and egoism. He is humble, unaffected by either
happiness or sorrow, and hasn't a single enemy. Greed, in-
justice, rashness, persecution of others, jealousy, stealing, harsh
words and cruelty are foreign to him. His heart is pure. He has
faith, innocence, simplicity and absolute truthfulness. By
Western norms he would be considered a saint, with this
addition: The Bhakti Yogi considers it as much a sin to waste
time as to waste talents—to him sins of omission are as great as
those of commission.

Finally we come to *Raja Yoga* which, translated literally,
means "King of Yogas." Raja Yoga takes its disciple through
eight stages, all of them highly spiritual and so complex we
shall not attempt to discuss any except the final one, *Samadhi*.
This is a state of bliss wherein the mind is withdrawn from
all earthly attachments. By then the Yogi has learned to stop
his thinking processes so completely that his consciousness is
absorbed into the Infinite. Just as a river flows inevitably to
the sea, so the individual mind merges into the ocean of Absolute
Consciousness. Those who have achieved Samadhi claim there
are no words to describe the experience—apparently it can
only be felt. In the state of Samadhi the Yogi sees without eyes,
tastes without tongue, hears without ears, smells without nose,
touches without contact. Sound and form are no more, suffering
and ignorance disappear, and the Yogi attains *Kaivalya* or
supreme liberation from earthly limitations. In this state, the
Yogi is supposedly able to free his astral body or etheric double

from his physical body. Raja Yoga may be thought of as the synthesis of all the systems of Yoga as a whole.

It is not vital to remember the various schools of Yoga or memorize the differences between them. Only the occasional reader will be tempted to try. What most persons will retain from this entire discussion is a "feel" of what it is about, and that is all that matters. Now to recapitulate: The gaining of a healthy body and a mind calm and passive under all circumstances is common to all Yogas. Control of one's mental processes as well as of the emotions is a basic common goal. This is achieved partly through conscious disciplines, partly by releasing the undercurrents of the mind at rest—or, to borrow psychological terminology, by giving play to the subconscious. In our own Occidental utilitarian terms, then, Yoga techniques, translated into *Yogism*, offer us the means for better Self-realization in the realm of the physical, the mental, the emotional and the spiritual. It is a royal road to inner power.

CHAPTER III

Physiological Aspects:
What Makes Yoga Possible

You have learned by now that there is nothing of magic in Yoga; neither are its results achieved magically, but by working for them. You have a good idea of its underlying philosophy, its scope and its application. You also know what you may and may not reasonably hope to gain from its study and practice, even within the limits of a form adapted to the exigencies of our busy, crowded, briskly-paced Western existence.

It goes without saying that such general knowledge would be of no use at all unless it went hand in hand with careful instruction. And, indeed, the major part of this book is therefore devoted to the specifics of Yoga practice. In Part II we shall take up, step by step, the minimal techniques which must be assimilated for complete body and mind control. Through these you will learn how to achieve true serenity of spirit and that mastery of Self which comes from self-knowledge, qualities developed by means of Yoga relaxation, concentration and meditation.

We have already pointed out that Yoga, in common with modern materialistic science, claims there is no artificial separation between that which is body and that which is mind, and that this is the logic behind the fact that all its teachings begin with the physical. Therefore to achieve the desired ends it becomes necessary to go through a process of re-educating the nerves, the muscles, the reflexes, until each part of the body is capable of controlling itself, utilizing its full reservoir of incipient power.

Naturally, however, busy men and women—for all their desire to function better—will not embark on such a program of self re-education nor subject themselves to self-discipline unless they thoroughly understand and accept the reasons for it. We are all human, and the tendency to shrug off whatever calls for even slight sustained effort is present in all of us. But we are generally willing to make that effort once we are convinced of its necessity, exactly as the mature student engineer is willing to study hard to master the basic rules of physics if he some day hopes to participate in building rockets.

Applied to the study of Yoga, what you need now is a thorough understanding of the relationship between the physiology of your body and the various exercises and poses whose practice Yoga calls for. Once this is clear, you will know exactly why you are being asked to do them and will be able to put your heart into the doing.

Try thinking of the body as a complex mechanism of which the skeleton is the marvelously flexible framework. There are over four hundred pair of muscles articulating this framework. There are parallel systems of nerves and blood vessels controlling its movements, its sensations, its responses; feeding it, cleaning it, replenishing it.

Some of the processes that comprise living are conscious, others automatic. Most of us, for instance, breathe without giving it a thought. Nor do we control the beating of the heart, or our digestive process, or our rate of metabolism. Nor, *until we have learned to be conscious of them*, are we even aware of the thousands of small motions we make in the course of the day, such as blinking, swallowing, shifting position while we think of ourselves as being reasonably still. In other words, we are making constant demands on our body before we even begin to use it for action.

In addition to bones, sinews and nerves, there is still another component in the picture we have sketched (p. 34)—one which medical science has only recently begun to know at all well—and that is the endocrine or ductless gland system. Since they are what makes all the other body functions possible, the endocrines may best be described as the power behind the throne. There are eight sets of endocrine glands in all: the pineal and the pituitary in the head; the thyroid, parathyroid

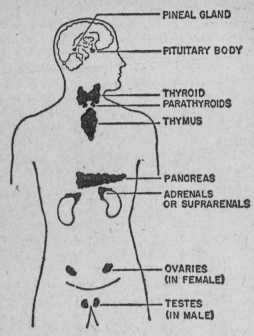

PINEAL GLAND

PITUITARY BODY

THYROID
PARATHYROIDS

THYMUS

PANCREAS

ADRENALS
OR SUPRARENALS

OVARIES
(IN FEMALE)

TESTES
(IN MALE)

and thymus in the region of the neck; the pancreas and the adrenals in the region of the solar plexus; and finally the gonads, or sex glands, in the pelvic region. Among them the endocrines control growth, weight, size, metabolism, energy, health, sexual power and even disposition. In short, they make us what we are.

When the Greeks taught that the seat of the emotions was the liver, they were not far from the truth. When Shakespeare wrote, "I have no stomach for it," he knew without benefit of X-ray that one's feelings, likes, and dislikes were closely bound up with what went on in the region of the solar plexus.

Today medical men ascertain the same thing with the use of barium and laboratory findings. But aren't they merely affirming, scientifically and accurately, what intuition and insight told wise men centuries ago?

In primitive man, as in animals, every adrenal upset served an immediate and useful purpose. Fear, alertness to danger, anger, hunger, the sex urge, all telegraphed their messages directly to the "stomach brain." The glands then sent their secretions into the blood stream, and the result was action. Primitive man, knowing fear, ran for safety. Knowing anger he struck out, or even killed. Feeling the urge to mate, he went wooing—even if he had to drag his bride home by the hair!

Today, with society and its laws sophisticated and complex, such simple cause-and-effect action and reaction is no longer possible. We have been taught to control, to hide, to sublimate, even to deny our emotions. Often we mask our impulses so completely we only know them translated into vague restlessness or sleeplessness or "butterflies in the stomach." They have become unrecognizable, but their basis remains the same: something—be it anger or fear or desire or pain—stimulates our endocrines; they respond, arouse our body, cause our heart to beat faster and our senses to quicken. But there is no physical outlet for all this turmoil. So the body turns upon itself. Literally, it is "spoiling" for action.

It is interesting that unlike our civilized consciousness the body and the subconscious have remained primitive. They cannot be easily fooled. Repressed emotions almost invariably become a weapon we turn against ourselves. If we worry, we lose weight—unless of course we happen to be among the compulsive eaters who gorge for consolation, in which case we gain alarmingly. If we get angry we find ourselves with an upset stomach, and if we stay angry long enough and frequently enough we may end up with colitis or ulcers. Overwhelmed by a sense of hopelessness, we may seek escape into asthma or tuberculosis or a state of shock. The list is endless. Each of us could add to it from personal observation.

Now add the problems imposed on us by our urban civilization: Our nervous system is called upon to work overtime
because of the endless stimuli coming at us relentlessly from
every direction. Among the tensions of city-living are street
noise, radio, TV, the telephone, crowds, work deadlines, demands on every minute of our time, constant distraction and,
of course, competitiveness. At best all this adds up to harass-
ment. Often anxieties are set up simply because of the pace we
try to keep up. Again the result is usually an upset of the deli-
cate balance of hormone secretions which are at the very basis
of our life force.

What it all adds up to is that most of us permit our minds
and our bodies to wage civil war upon each other instead of
having them unite to serve us, and serve us well.

Clearly, then, the problem is to put our own selves in control.

Just how does the practice of Yoga, with its breathing
exercise and formal postures, help to achieve this? On what
physiological principles can it be said to base itself? Here are
some of the answers the student should have before becoming
more deeply involved.

First the physiology of breathing:

The purpose of breathing, as everyone knows, is to supply
the body with oxygen and cleanse it of carbon dioxide. Cut
off the oxygen, retain the poisonous waste gas, and death will
follow in a matter of minutes. This is elementary. What is not
so clear is that an *inadequate* supply of oxygen—that is, improper waste disposal—results in half-living. The body functions are slowed, the tissues fail to renew themselves. Yet this
unsatisfactory state of affairs is so common that we actually
take it for granted. In fact, leading chest specialists say that the
average person today utilizes only about one-eighth of his
lung capacity, a capacity which was right for him back in the
days when he lived in caves and spent all his waking hours
actively engaged in the business of surviving.

Even when we are not living at par, the heart does a prodi-
gious job. Every hour it pumps some 800 quarts of blood

through the lungs which, in turn, eliminate some 30 quarts of carbon acid during that time. The heart beats 100,000 times a day, which means it generates enough energy to lift a weight of 130 tons a foot high. It pumps enough blood in a lifetime to float the largest ocean liner. Imagine what power our heart might have, what energy it could generate, if only its supply of oxygen were increased eight times!

As the freshly-oxygenated blood travels from the lungs to the heart and is pumped on, via arteries and blood vessels, via tiny capillaries, it reaches every cell in our organism. It makes possible the utilization of our food intake for the body's various needs, rebuilding tissues, supplying energy. It stimulates the functioning of the endocrine glands so that their secretions may be better absorbed. It feeds the nerves. It feeds the brain. Then, through a second set of capillaries, dark red now instead of bright, for it is loaded with waste, it travels back through the veins to be cleansed once more. All of the blood in the body makes this trip to the heart every three minutes.

Now what of the lungs? Why is it that most of us do not use our respiratory system properly? Partly the answer is, again, that we have grown effete with civilization. The physiology of the human body remains geared to that primitive state when man hunted, climbed trees, split rocks, and there is little we can do to change this. In a sense we now have too much equipment for our needs, and we are letting it grow weak and flabby with disuse. This imbalance, by the way, has been largely responsible for the prevalence of tuberculosis and our susceptibility to it until the development of wonder drugs changed the picture.

But the anachronistic way we are built is not the only reason for our being oxygen-starved, nor for the various respiratory ailments and infection from which so many of us suffer. The fact is, few of us breathe properly.

Look around you. You will be astonished to notice how many people breathe through the mouth instead of through the nose. This means they inhale directly through the pharynx and the larynx (roughly, together, the throat) allowing air to reach the bronchial tubes without being properly filtered and warmed. In order to be cleansed of dust and bacteria air should be drawn in through the nasal passages where the mucous membranes with their secretions filter it. Moreover, as that air then travels a considerably longer road it is warmed to body temperature instead of being allowed to hit vital organs with chilly shock. Breathing through the mouth, then, is an invitation to colds and infections of all sorts.

One final aspect, too often disregarded, of proper breathing is that it must be done from the diaphragm. Women especially, because of tight clothing and girdles, tend to breathe by lifting the chest, consciously drawing the air in. This is less than half-effective, both because the upper lobes of the lungs are the smallest and because the upper part of the rib cage is relatively rigid. The correct way to breathe is to expand the muscles of the diaphragm down and out, then push in and up. In this way the lungs expand to full capacity, air rushes into them, then is vigorously expelled. If you try it, you will quickly see how even a minute or two of such breathing can be enormously exhilarating. But very few of us breathe this way naturally. It is something which must be learned by practice.

Yoga deep-breathing exercises, as you will see shortly, give the body this exhilaration. Some you will find extremely simple —so simple you will wonder why they should be dignified by such formal attention. The answer is that because of this very simplicity they can, if done regularly, soon become automatic, a fine new habit. Moreover, like the more complicated ones, they are a most important adjunct of the practice of relaxation and concentration. Bear in mind always that one cannot be achieved without the other, and neither can be reached without an understanding of the purpose of both.

Try this first experiment in Dynamic Breathing: Stand straight but relaxed. Breathing as smoothly and rhythmically as possible, with the mouth closed, inhale slowly and deeply while expanding the diaphragm, then exhale by pushing the diaphragm in and up. Take as long to inhale as to exhale, although normally inhalation involves a shorter movement than exhalation. While striving to equalize and slow down your normal tempo, visualize your limbs as hollow tubes through which the life-giving *prana* is being drawn into your body. Picture this energy flowing into your organs, bathing your entire body and cleansing it. As you exhale, visualize fatigue and exhaustion passing out of your system along with the poisonous wastes you breathe out. Finish with what we call the "Cleansing Breath:" Inhale deeply, then, when your lungs are fully extended, expel the breath suddenly and energetically, using a quick inward jerk of the abdomen to drain the lungs of all air. Repeat the cleansing breath two or three times, and you will be amazed at its bracing effect. After you have become expert at Dynamic Breathing, you can practice it at odd times during the day.

Now for the physiology of relaxation and concentration:

On the face of it, talking about the physiology of mental attitudes may sound odd. It isn't, when you give it thought. But perhaps the concept of a purely physical aspect of what we habitually consider primarily mental states will become clearer if we stop to analyze their opposites—nervous tension and the inability to concentrate.

Do you remember being told, back when you were very young and frightened and facing a Big Moment, to take a deep breath, count to ten, then plunge ahead? What was *that* if not a time-honored trick for achieving relaxation through breathing? The young actor is advised to do this; so is the inexperienced public speaker—while the experienced ones do it almost as a reflex.

The Yoga sages discovered thousands of years ago that in order to gain complete control of the body and thus free the mind, it was imperative to get more out of the organs than is generally considered possible. We have just seen how correct breathing contributes to this. Next let us analyze relaxation itself and find out something about the positions the body needs to assume in order to relax. Let us also see how relaxation really is possible in postures which, to our Western eye, look like tortured contortions.

Phrased another way, what is the relationship between the Yoga positions, the *asanas* and *mudras*, and the physical as well as mental results claimed for them? Why is it so important to follow these routines? Why, in short, can't we simply relax in the old, orthodox way, slumped in a chair or lying in bed?

In the first place, there probably never was any such thing as an old, orthodox method of relaxation. Try to check on yourself and you will begin at once to see the fallacies: Slump in an armchair, and you will find you retain tensions in a dozen muscles. Are you frowning, grinding your teeth, drumming your fingers on the arm of the chair, tapping your foot? Is the back of your neck tight? Are you keenly aware of every sound around you? Check closely, and you will be astonished at what you discover.

Now try lying flat on the floor a few moments. Close your eyes, let your arms and legs go limp, your neck and spine loose. Can you tell the difference? Of course you can. Tension begins to flow out of you almost at once, yet you haven't even learned how to lie down *properly*.

The principles of relaxation on which all *asanas* are based are these: It is essential to find positions in which it is possible to "let go" as many muscles as possible and as many thoughts as possible. This relieves both mind and body of all conscious tension and contraction. Naturally total relaxation is not possible, especially in a seated position, for in order to hold the back erect certain muscles must of necessity remain contracted. But if the body is balanced and at ease, very little effort is required to keep it erect. This balance and limberness of muscle is what the Yogi develops through assiduous practice.

It is a mistake to assume, by the way, as some students do, that in order to be successful, *asanas* must be hard to do. Many are simple enough for anyone to assimilate comfortably; others, while difficult at first, soon respond to steady, patient application. Moreover, rather than risk discouragement the Occidental is always advised to start out with a preliminary series of easy, comfortable stretching exercises.

Conscious stretching, together with conscious relaxation, are the best possible preliminaries to the practice of *asanas*. Their techniques are given in detail in Part II of this book, but right now try a few simple routines:

After you have completed your Dynamic Breathing and the Cleansing Breath, stand straight but relaxed and slowly start to bend over so that your fingers touch your toes. Begin by relaxing your neck so that your chin touches your chest, let the chest cave in while the shoulders move forward and your arms hang loose and limp. Arch your spine and try to bend, vertebra by vertebra in a rolling motion until your whole torso feels limp like the body of a rag doll. If you cannot touch your toes the first time, do not strain to do it; instead, try to bend lower by pushing the body from the waist down in a few easy, jerking motions. Now straighten up by reversing the process—tense each vertebra in turn, this time from the waist up. Now do a thorough stretch, breathing deeply and luxuriously. Repeat once or twice. You will be astonished at the elasticity your spine acquires if you do this regularly every day for a week.

Another excellent preliminary relaxation routine is stretching on waking up. Make it a habit never to jump out of bed in the morning. Instead, give yourself a minute or two to wake your body thoroughly. Lie flat on your back, preferably without a pillow. Breathing deeply but easily, start by consciously stretching one leg from the hip down, toes pointing so that you can feel the muscles of the calf, and the leg itself feels about an inch longer than the other. Relax, then repeat with the other leg. Now stretch your arms hard sideways, then over your head, tensing shoulder and neck and muscles, and arching your back like a cat. Now get up *slowly*, avoiding jerky motions. You have never seen a dog or cat jump up from a nap, unless it has been startled and alerted as if to danger, in which case its adrenalin is probably pouring through its body. It is precisely such harmful purposeless over-stimulation that you must teach yourself to avoid. Incidentally, this getting-up routine is worth an extra half hour's sleep.

We have already mentioned that the ancient Yogis developed their exercise techniques from observing animal life. Not only did they appreciate the genius for relaxation all animals possess. They realized that animals, utilizing their energies properly, sleeping at intervals around the clock, eating only according to need, live to five times their maturity and keep their full vigor five-sixths of their life, while men and women live to only twice their maturity and begin to lose their vitality half-way through. Carrying their emulation of beasts and birds to a logical conclusion the Yogis became the exception to the rule. Highly cultivated, highly civilized as they are, they know enough to turn to the simple and the primitive in order to re-discover natural living and nature's laws.

Obviously the pursuit of the art of relaxation isn't a matter of physical positions alone. Since relaxation is a matter for the mind and spirit as well as for the body, other factors too are involved and they will be discussed at the proper time. But while we are still on the physiological aspects, it should be pointed out that, like proper breathing, correct posture sets up the ideal conditions for the mental and spiritual side of Yoga, since in a relaxed body the blood, stimulated by greater amounts of oxygen, flushes poisons out of every cell. This results in a greater sense of well-being, the body becoming alert, magnificently responsive to the dictates of mind and of will. Thus the Yogi may then be likened to a consummate artist capable of drawing the best out of a perfect, responsive instrument.

The more completely you learn to control the body the more of its various functions become controllable. For instance, with the mind at peace the great Western bugaboo of insomnia quickly vanishes. Not only does sleep begin to come easily to the person who practices Yoga—its very quality is different—sleep that is deep, calm, profoundly dreamless and restful.

As the tone of the body improves and rest becomes more thorough, metabolism too begins to improve. There is less need for food, since whatever food is taken in is digested and utilized to the last molecule. Hence weight problems begin to disappear.

The overweight see their fat burn away while the under-weight begin to gain as food begins to do them some good. Next the body, physiologically on its toes, is able to throw off infection, sore throats, migraine and the many ailments of creeping middle age. Specifically the whole gamut of joint diseases such as arthritis, rheumatism and neuritis recede under the double offensive of improved circulation and gently-limbering exercise.

In India it is not at all uncommon to meet Yogis a hundred years old and older. These men, after years of study and con-centration, often are capable of amazing feats. It is not rare to hear of long fasts, of breathing so controlled it approaches what in the animal world is called a state of hibernation. Yogis often also develop total indifference to pain. The men who lie on beds of nails, who allow themselves to be buried alive for days on end, may be fakirs but not necessarily fakers. It has been done, and will be done many times again. For what they have developed is the ability to exist in a state of suspended animation.

Naturally, this book cannot be expected to teach the Wester-ner any such refinements of performance. Aside from the dangers we have already mentioned, it is doubtful that most students would be interested. Rather let us decide soberly and realistically on a modest program of attainment which, just as a beginning, might include the triple goal of greater peace of mind, greater self-knowledge and improved health. If we do that much we may find ourselves, in a surprisingly short time, embarking on second youth—a youth made joyous by added wisdom, a new-found serenity and, consequently, happier relationships with those around us. Best of all, these goals may be achieved within the limited time we have at our disposal, with only a reasonable store of patience and well within the scope of activities of our everyday life.

CHAPTER IV

Yoga, Medicine and Psychiatry

Shortly after World War II a team of UNESCO health experts were visiting the Balkans. A woman doctor stopped to talk about mother-and-child problems to a group of peasant women in a Bulgarian village. One of the young mothers, a lusty girl in her middle twenties, turned out to be the bride of the most important man in the community—a great oak of a man past ninety. The girl had felt highly honored when, having buried his fourth wife, the local bigwig had chosen her from among his neighbors' marriageable daughters to be Number Five. Now she was proudly showing off her son, born exactly nine months after the wedding. As the doctor told it afterwards, there was no doubt as to family resemblance. The child was a miniature replica of his father.

Startled, the doctor tried, as tactfully as she could, to draw the girl out. After all, she hinted, woman-to-woman, the man had grandsons older than the bride. Was there, perhaps, some tribal custom about stand-ins . . .

The girl seemed puzzled and in the end the doctor asked her question more plainly. Did the nonagenarian really still want sex? The girl's amazement showed in her face. Of course! Otherwise what would he want with a wife? Was the doctor trying to say that in other parts of the world things were different?

Granted these rugged mountaineers, raised on mare's milk and goat cheese, are an exception even in their own country. Still the story suggests interesting speculation. Since the village apparently had never heard of impotence as a must for its senior citizens, might it not follow that, conditioned neither to fear nor even to expect it, the men simply did not succumb to it?

The next question to ask ourselves is, inevitably, this: How often do we succumb to illness, weariness, and especially the creeping symptoms of old age, largely because that is the pattern we have been taught to envisage? *Youth is a state of the soul,* someone once said. Youth is also a state of the spirit, a state of mind, a state of the glands. It is a matter of the way the heart beats and the reflexes function. No one can hope to feel young if he is self-engrossed to the point of being the center of his universe. Now broaden this concept to encompass general well-being: again it is a matter of outlook—we feel as we have been conditioned to feel.

Think of various persons you have known. Frail or vigorous, those you remember with pleasure are the ones whose spirit is in command, who can shrug off disappointment or misfortune or even pain not because of some absurd Pollyanna mechanism or because they enjoy being martyrs, but because they have a sense of proportion—they never bog down. To such people enslavement by the body or by purely personal considerations is inconceivable. They can see well beyond themselves, hence they are free and well-adjusted human beings who remain on good terms with Time.

Western civilization has for centuries laid so much stress on the individual and his happiness that more than any other group on earth we tend to allow ourselves to feel overwhelmed when personal happiness is lacking. We also tend to set up romantic goals, forever striving toward some perfect ending without end, then feeling devastated because life doesn't work that way. Hence the enormous discrepancy between our dreams and our realities, hence endless worry, tension and discontent.

Eastern philosophies in general take a vastly different view. The individual counts for less and therefore expects less from life; to put it another way, he neither starts out feeling as important to himself as we do, nor does he lay himself open to as much disappointment. In other words, he starts out with more of a sense of proportion about himself and his relationship to the cosmic whole. Yoga puts great stress on this.

Whether this is a better orientation than ours or one not as happy is beside the point. The fact remains that such a philosophy does keep the individual from being prey to the restlessness, unhappiness and hidden fears which help destroy us.

Our Western preoccupation with Self has for a long time been yielding bitter fruit. Among our neurotic Victorian grandparents it was the common thing for ladies to have the vapors and to faint dead away, and both women and strong men "took to their bed" when they felt powerless to cope with problems. Today, with medical science more probing and diagnosis more exact, we no longer fool ourselves with such simple tactics. Escape into illness has to take more subtle forms. It does. Needless to say the long list of disorders classed as psychogenic proves that it remains equally effective.

Our other way of expressing frustration is through mental disturbance of varying intensity and depth. (By this we mean psychiatric and psychological upsets as differentiated from mental illness of physical origin). Today in the United States about fifty percent of all hospital beds are occupied by mental patients. This is a staggering statistic made all the more formidable by doctors' statements about how many would-be patients remain undiagnosed. In addition we all know that every psychoanalyst, every psychiatrist setting up in practice throughout the country has more patients than he can handle. From this we must conclude that our unhappiness quotient has become the highest in the world. Yet ours is also the country with the highest standard of living, the highest per capita income, the most luxuries. Obviously something is seriously out of kilter somewhere.

The Yogi would tell us that we permit ourselves to be ruled and torn, looking for happiness outside rather than within. We do not clearly understand the difference between shadow and substance. We wear ourselves down with our unquiet.

Now let us listen to the anguished cry of the patient who seeks the help of an analyst: What is he after as he lies down on the green couch? Here again the overall, meaningless answer is happiness. Pinpointed, this means peace of mind, a sense of balance, a sense of belonging, the ability to live with himself and with others.

The analyst listens with an objectivity to which he has been trained, then slowly tries to help the patient see himself objectively too. This generally turns out to be a slow, difficult process; the cost, in financial as well as emotional disbursement, exhorbitant. It often takes years to re-educate and reorient the psyche, largely because we all resist honest insights which are apt to be both unflattering and painful.

The patient study of Yoga can often produce the same results much more quickly and at less cost. But the path of attainment is very different indeed.

Here, however, it is important to make very clear to the reader that we are not counter-posing the two methods on an either-or basis. Certainly it would be both dangerous and fool-hardy, if you were feeling ill, to decide for yourself whether or not your symptoms were real or mentally-induced. Such decisions are best left to a competent doctor. The same holds true for cases of severe mental stress; it would be throwing out the baby with the bath to turn one's back on techniques which modern science has made available to us. Remember, *Yoga does not decry medicine*. It does not turn its back on plain common sense. Certainly it is not a form of faith healing. But it has its own ways of dealing with inner turmoil which, for want of a more concrete name, we might call soul-sickness. Over the centuries it has discovered and learned to utilize age-old truths and a combined knowledge of body and mind which modern medicine and Sigmund Freud have only recently concretized for the West.

Do not think that even in India the path of the Yogi disciple, the *Chela*, is easy. We are told that often people seek out a personal Guru not for wisdom, but in order to gratify some inner weakness. They want him for the purpose of self-escape. They hope to pass on to him their own burden of cares or responsibilities, thereby making life simple and easy, precisely as some Westerners seek a father-confessor and others an analyst. But neither in the West nor in the East is there any easy road to wisdom.

Like the patient on the couch, the student of Yoga makes progress only as he takes upon himself alone the responsibility for learning. Unlike the man or woman in analysis, he starts with the physical, then progresses to controlling the mind. Take as an example the basic exercises in concentration and the way these may eventually be utilized for self-knowledge.

A typical exercise is to sit on the floor, tailor fashion, choose a mental target of the simplest kind—a spot on the wall before you, a piece of paper, your own nose—and concentrate on that target for thirty seconds. You may close your eyes and continue visualizing it until you lose it—and lose it you will—then open your eyes and capture it again.

This may seem absurdly easy—until you try it. Few of us realize how our minds are apt to flit from thought to thought and how much discipline it takes to conquer this tendency. It does little good to be stern and make good resolutions about self-control. They won't work. What will work, however, is steady, repeated, conscious practice. At the end of a few weeks the daily thirty seconds' concentration stint may even be stretched to a whole minute. You will be surprised how long the minute lasts.

Now consider the many ways in which developing your power to concentrate can benefit you in your search for self-knowledge. We all know how quickly, how instinctively we shy away from unpleasant thoughts, especially if these thoughts happen to be directed against ourselves. Yet in order to learn to know ourselves it is essential to turn on the searchlight of the mind and survey without turning away or glossing over whatever we find inside, unattractive and unflattering as the discovery may be.

One reason why self-analysis is all but impossible for the average person is because such sustained examination is in itself all but impossible. We may start out with every intention of being objective and ruthlessly honest, but when the going gets tough our mind will play tricks on us. All at once we will find ourselves thinking, not of the facet of our personality we have just discovered we do not like, but of how interestingly that same weakness colors the behavior of a friend, and how understanding we have been of the friend in a time of need, and why didn't we get more appreciation, anyway? Once the chain of association starts, there is no stopping it.

A basic exercise in concentration, however, can serve to break the habit of flitting until we have learned to stay with the thought we have chosen. In this way it becomes the key—or rather, one of the many keys—to mastering the art of self-analysis.

Another striking parallel between the analytical method and Yoga practice is in the realm of dreams. In a general way everyone is now familiar with the use analysis makes of dream material. Yoga, on the other hand, makes it possible to control dreams until they flow in orderly fashion, are remembered and provide revealing insights; this the advanced student can accomplish by *willing* himself to dream, just as he can will himself to go to sleep and wake up at a certain time. He can thus make the subconscious work subliminally, to good advantage, while the conscious mind rests.

But perhaps the most important contribution to self-knowledge, and the one which can do most toward freeing you of anxiety, is that as you practice concentration and relaxation exercises, as your thoughts learn to flow where you direct them, you will gain a deep awareness of who you are. Without becoming either detached or indifferent, you will nevertheless learn to detach yourself from your surroundings enough to no longer feel constantly and closely identified with everything that happens around you. You will be able to do this for the simple reason that you will no longer have the same need to lean. You will have found strength within yourself to be yourself. You will be able to meet the world on your own terms, on a basis of maturity and independence. And that, above all, means getting the very best out of yourself.

PART II

THE PRACTICE OF YOGA

*How You Can Benefit in Many Ways
From Daily Use of Yoga Techniques*

CHAPTER V

Pranayama: The Breath of Life

The air we breathe is the only element our body cannot do without for even the shortest time. We can, if necessary, survive without food for as long as a month, without water for many days. But deprive the body of oxygen and we die within minutes. Cut off the supply of oxygen to the brain, and vital tissues are permanently destroyed.

Thousands of years ago the Hindee had come to understand the importance of breath so thoroughly that we find the following legend told in one of their oldest scriptures, the *Brihadaranyaka Upanishad*:

"The senses, quarrelling amongst themselves one day as to who was the best, went to Brahma and said, 'Who is the richest of us—tell us!' And Brahma replied, 'He by whose departure the body seems worst, he is the richest.' And they determined to find out.

"First the eye departed, and having been absent a year it came back, asking, 'How have you been able to live without me?' They replied, 'Like blind people, not seeing with the eye, but breathing with the breath, speaking with the tongue, hearing with the ear, knowing with the mind, generating with the seed. Thus have we lived.' And the eye returned to its place.

"Next the ear departed, and at the end of a year it came back, asking the same question. And they replied, 'Like deaf people have we lived, not hearing with the ear, but breathing with the breath, speaking with the tongue, seeing with the eye, knowing with the mind, generating with the seed.' And the ear returned to its place.

"Next it was the turn of the mind, and after it had been gone a year, and returned, they said, 'We have lived like fools without you, but we have lived.' And to the seed, after it had been gone a year, they said, 'We have lived like impotent people, but we have lived.' And the mind and the seed each returned to his place.

"And now it was the turn of the breath. And on the point of departing it tore up the other senses, as a great excellent horse of the Sindhu country might tear up the pegs to which he is tethered. Then all the other senses called out to him, 'Sir, do not leave us! We shall not be able to live without thee'!"

Is it not surprising that this ancient parable coincides with scientific truth? The first step toward re-orienting and improving the functioning of your mind and body is learning to utilize—really utilize—the air you breathe. The Yogis were the first to discover the importance of this and so actually devised an exact science of breathing. They called it PRANAYAMA, from the Sanskrit word *prana*, meaning breath, and *yama*, its cessation. They also explored *pranayama* from every point of view—the practical and physiological and also the mystical—for to them breathing was much more than just one of the necessary body processes.

First let us consider the purely physical side of breathing:

Air is nourishment to our bodies just as much as food and drink. Air gives our blood stream the supply of oxygen it must have in order to feed itself so that it may, in turn, feed the tissues, nerves, glands and vital organs. Without it our skin, bones, teeth and hair could not remain in condition. Our digestion—the process of utilizing the food we eat—fails at once without a proper supply of oxygen to the blood. Even our thinking processes are slowed down without intake and exhalation of fresh air—which is the reason mental sluggishness overtakes us in an ill-ventilated room. Some authorities have even come to believe there is a direct relationship between a child's I.Q. and the supply of oxygen in its system—a low I.Q. being often traceable to bad posture, adenoids or merely bad breathing habits. Change these, and a sluggish youngster often blossoms overnight into a bright, responsive one!

To function properly, the brain needs three times more oxygen than the rest of our organs; and unless this is provided it will try to appropriate its supply by drawing on the overall allotment. This explains why so many city people, working at sedentary jobs, "using their heads," so to speak, all day long, tend to become debilitated and have greater susceptibility to germs and infections than persons who lead active outdoor lives. Sedentary individuals are permanently oxygen-starved. Yet this situation can be avoided at will, as this chapter will show you.

In a single day we breathe about 23,000 times. The average volume of air taken in with a single breath is about 20 cubic inches, depending on a person's size, sex, posture, the nature of the surrounding atmosphere and one's physical and emotional state. However, with proper attention given to the breathing act, this volume may be increased to 100 or even 130 cubic inches per breath. In other words, careful re-orientation of your habits can provide you with five times the oxygen, and rid you of five times the carbon dioxide, with which you habitually function.

In Chapter III we dwelt very briefly on the physiology of breathing. Here is what takes place during the breathing process: When you breathe properly—that is, with the mouth closed so that the air is inhaled through the nasal passages—oxygen travels down the pharynx (rear of the throat), the larynx (roughly the region of the Adam's apple), and the trachia or windpipe until it reaches the bronchial tubes. By then most of the dust and bacteria have been filtered out by the mucous membranes, or the moist lining of the nose. Mucous, by the way, in addition to acting as a filter substance, also has certain germicidal properties—another reason why it is so important to cultivate the habit of breathing through the nose, never through the mouth. A third reason, already mentioned elsewhere, is that while traveling this somewhat longer road the air is warmed to proper body temperature, which means extra insurance against catching colds.

After having been thus filtered and warmed, the supply of air moves on from the bronchiae into the lungs. Here it enters millions of cells—600,000,000 of them to be exact, if you can visualize such an astronomic figure—each of which is a tiny air sac. Surrounding these is a network of equally tiny blood vessels or capillaries. The blood absorbs the fresh oxygen directly through the cell walls at the same time as it rids itself of the carbon dioxide from the last trip.

Next the freshly oxygenated blood travels to the heart. The heart pumps it via arteries and blood vessels to every part of the body, where in turn it seeps into every tissue and bone cell. In this manner 800 quarts of blood pass through the heart and lungs every hour. Small wonder, then, that the condition of your heart so closely governs your life expectancy!

By now it should be amply clear why both a proper technique of breathing and the quality of the air we take in are of such vital importance to our general health. The Yogis were aware of this long before the British scientist Harvey, in the seventeenth century, formulated the first facts about blood circulation for us in the Western hemisphere! But they also knew something else: Not only does *pranayama* help keep the human body healthy; it helps it stay youthful, supple, slim and vital, and for the following obvious reasons:

As the average person reaches middle age, lung tissues tend to grow less and less elastic. Years of improper breathing take their toll. The chest itself has a tendency to grow rigid. The consequence is an accumulation of uric acid in the blood stream which often leads to any one of those somewhat vague syndromes of pain and discomfort that doctors in general diagnose with a shrug as the miseries of aging, which they cheerfully advise you to learn to live with since nothing can be done about them. Backaches, headaches, stiffening muscles and joints, neuritis, rheumatism are some of the more common of these complaints. Excess fat is another, for as we begin to grow old and proper circulation is impeded by a sluggish diaphragm or hardening arteries, the red blood corpuscles become distributed unevenly and fat accumulates in spots instead of being burned up. Yet all of these complaints may be avoided, or at least considerably retarded, if only we learn to breathe scientifically. In the case of obesity, which of course can be further countered by some of the Yoga "contraction" exercises to be discussed later on, deep breathing itself has a direct salutary effect on it. For the cleansing, stimulating action of deep breathing improves metabolism and that, in turn, transforms deposits of fat into body fuel, or added energy.

So much, then, for the physiology of breath. But *pranayama* is not physical breathing alone. Nor is *prana* to be confused with air. It is a far more subtle substance. Without going too deeply into Yogi metaphysical concepts, let us try to arrive at an understanding of it in terms acceptable to us Western materialists.

A century before the scientists Priestley and Lavoisier conducted their famous experiments isolating oxygen as the substance which made air all-important to life, a British chemist named Maynow ran a series of tests, revolutionary for his times, which convinced him that life was supported "not by air alone but by a more active and subtle part of it." He went so far as to suggest that the lungs were the organ which separated this substance from the atmosphere and passed it into the blood. This substance, or rather this hidden property in the atmosphere, he called *spiritus igneo-aereus*, and excitedly presented a paper on it to his fellow-members in the Royal Society. But because in mid-seventeenth century the accepted medical belief was that the purpose of breathing was "to cool the heart," Maynow's learned colleagues held him up to ridicule. His theory was most effectively buried.

The Hindu theory of *prana* goes much further than Maynow's intuitive reasoning. We might paraphrase it by saying that oxygen itself is the overall stream within which flows a far more subtle force about which we Occidentals know all too little; nor have we ever paid much attention to it inasmuch as no instruments have yet been invented with which to measure and define it. (No need here to dwell on how skeptical we in this part of the world tend to be of whatever cannot be explained away in purely materialistic terms!) Yet whether we like it or not this force seems to exist just the same—a latent vital power ready to be harnessed for our benefit if we so desire. In fact, the Hindee believe that *all* physical and mental manifestations are dependent upon *prana*. They call it the breath of life. Another definition of it is Absolute, or Cosmic energy, and it may help your concept of it if you think of *pranayama* as the means for filling the physical body with this cosmic energy.

The Yogis say that *prana* circulates through the human body via a network of special channels called *nadis*, roughly equivalent to our network of nerves and blood vessels. The nadis, in turn, are governed by seven *chakras*, or wheels, which roughly are the astral counterparts of our anatomic plexuses (see pages 58-59). The three main nadis are called *Ida*, *Pingala* and *Shushamna*. Shushamna corresponds to the spinal cord, while Ida and Pingala are represented as two intercircling snakes on either side of it and may be identified with the sympathetic nervous system.

Of the chakras, the lowest, *Muladhara*, is situated at the base of the spine, corresponding to the sacral plexus. At the physical level it is said to control the process of elimination. But it is also a most important center for controlling the dormant energy called *Kundalini*, or the Serpent Power already mentioned in Chapter II. This, when released, brings with it among other things the knowledge of good and evil. In modern Western terms Kundalini may be said to control the deepest aspects of the personality, most especially the subconscious. Probably the closest analogy in terms of our own concepts would be that what Freud calls the *libido*—man's deepest sex drive which, sublimated, translates itself into the source of all creative, emotional and spiritual drives.

The second chakra, *Svadishthana*, situated in the region of the genitals, is said to control overt sexual desire. Next comes *Manipura*, which corresponds to the solar plexus, with control over the digestive processes. This is the "stomach brain," our powerhouse of stored-up energy in many ways connected with all manner of physical reactions and emotions. The fourth chakra, *Anahat*, at heart level, corresponds to the cardiac plexus, which controls breathing. The fifth is the *Visuadha*, behind the throat, which controls speech. The sixth, *Ajna*, located between the eyebrows, supposedly controls the autonomous nervous system and is said to be the seat of the mystical "third eye" which accounts for the clairvoyance claimed by some Yogis. Finally there is *Sahasrara* chakra, called also the Thousand-Petalled Lotus, which corresponds to the cortical layer of the brain. Of this Chakra it is said that here Kundalini joins her Lord, Vishnu, as matter ascends to the spirit and the gross in the human body merges with what is most lofty.

The mystical ramifications of this concept need not concern us here, but whatever the differences between prana and oxygen, one thing is certain: the practice of *pranayama*—even if you are determined to call it simply proper breathing—produces immediate beneficial results. In short order the student begins to experience lightness of body, an absence of restlessness, better digestion due to an increase in the flow of the gastric juices, clearing and smoothing of the skin. The physiological benefits we have already explained—now let the student discover for himself how *quickly* these will come to him once he establishes a daily routine of exercises. As for the spiritual well-being that will follow—the inner lightness, the serenity—it matters little whether you attribute them to oxygen burning out the wastes and poisons in your grey matter or to more subtle influences. The important thing is that it is all yours to enjoy at will.

And now for method:

Except for certain exercises which specify otherwise, breathing, as you now know, should always be through the nose. It should also be rhythmic. A long inhalation, a short pause while holding the breath, then a long exhalation is the basic pattern to follow. But on no account must you make hard work of it or overdo it. Strain destroys the benefits of the exercise. And regardless of what you may have heard about suspension of breath practiced by some Yogis, this is nothing for a neophyte to experiment with. In fact, it might be harmful. So the moment you feel the least bit queer when practicing Yogic breathing, stop.

This deep rhythmic breathing, for which a few simple exercises follow, is not to be confused with the kind of *effortless dynamic breathing* which you should also learn, then assimilate so completely that you will be doing it unconsciously all the time. Most of us breathe in short staccato jerks, shallowly, aimlessly. If for a while you take time to watch yourself, if you train yourself to breathe more slowly and more deeply, though without the pause between inhalation and exhalation as recommended for special exercises, the new rhythm will shortly become automatic. From about fifteen breaths a minute —or 21,600 each twenty-four hours—you will have reduced your tempo by possibly three breaths a minute, which is twenty percent, or 4,320 per day. Such a slowing-down means a corresponding easing of the wear-and-tear on the entire body —less work for the heart, lower blood pressure, a relaxation of body tensions, and quieter nerves—in short, still another way to lengthen the years of your life and make them enjoyable!

Of all the Yoga exercises and poses, the breathing routines are done with least effort. They take very little time and may be done anywhere, just as effortless Dynamic Breathing may be practiced while you go out for a walk or sit in an easy chair to rest. So even if you have no time for any of the routines discussed in other chapters, under no circumstances omit your deep breathing, regardless of how crowded your schedule or how long your day.

The following deep-breathing exercises are most effective if done upon arising. They are best performed before an open window but may also be practiced before going to bed or even sometime during the day.

Stand erect and at ease. Place the hands on the hips, elbows well out and never forced backward. Draw the chest straight upward, then press the hip bones with the hands in a downward direction. By this means a vacuum will be formed and air will rush into the lungs of its own accord. Remember to keep the nostrils wide open so that the nose may serve as a passive channel for inhaling and exhaling. The breathing should be noiseless. Remember to stretch the upper part of the trunk. The chest must never be cramped, the abdomen should be naturally relaxed, the spine and neck straight. Remember not to draw the abdomen inward; lift the shoulders up, never force them back.

To exhale, allow the ribs of the upper part of the trunk to sink down gradually. Then lift the lower ribs and abdomen slowly. Again, care must be taken not to bend the body or arch the chest. Exhale silently through the mouth. At first do not retain the breath after inhalation. Start with three or four rounds a day; increase by one each week.

An excellent way to practice *pranayama* is lying down. Lie flat on a hard surface—preferably on the floor, using a mat or rug. Let your arms rest by your sides, parallel to the body. Keep the legs straight but not stiff. Relax muscles and mind, step by step, as in Savasana, the exercise for complete relaxation (Chapter VI). Breathe deeply and noiselessly from the diaphragm. Start with three or four rounds a day, increasing by one round each week. This exercise may be done in conjunction with complete relaxation, but do not substitute one for the other. Also, do not try to use a bed unless it is an exceptionally hard one, since relaxing on a hard surface is by far the most effective method.

Persons engaged in sedentary occupations will derive great benefit from practicing *pranayama* while sitting comfortably upright in an easy chair. For this exercise, inhale through both nostrils, then hold the breath for a short time before exhaling effortlessly. No strict ratio need be established between inhalation, retention and exhalation so long as the process is deep and natural. The important thing is that rhythm be established in the entire being, so that the nerves are toned and the mind calmed. You will be astonished how much easier your next task of studying or working will become, how unrest and disturbing elements will vanish from your consciousness. Fatigue will disappear and you will feel deeply refreshed. However, in order to get the full benefit of this exercise you must remember to keep not only your body but your mind

passive. Try to blank out all conscious thought, concentrating
—as you breathe—on some bland, pleasing object directly before your eyes.

Controlling mental images during the practice of *pranayama*
is a conscious discipline which must be learned. The average
person's mind, left to itself, dances like a flame in the wind.
It flits from image to image, free-associating, as the psychiatrists
call it, allowing full play to the imagination, to day-dreaming, to
wishful thinking. With the mind racing this way, no true
relaxation or meditation is possible. The Yogis devised the
following exercise to counteract this tendency to wool-gather:

Stare steadily and without blinking at some small object
directly in your line of vision. Continue until tears begin to
form in your eyes. You need not be alarmed at the slight sting-
ing sensation you will have—there is nothing harmful to the
sight here; on the contrary, your eyes will be strengthened. At
the same time you will be developing will power. (The Yogis
claim this exercise is an early step to clairvoyance, but of course
this is not an area we propose to explore in this book.) If your
sight is poor or your eyes tire easily, try the following routine
after the concentration routine: While breathing slowly inward, roll the eyes with a circular motion outward; then exhale,
rolling the eyes inward. Repeat three times, then reverse, and
rest.

Once you have mastered the technique of *pranayama*, you
may go on to other breathing exercises for further strengthening the body. Here are a few:

Sitkari, the first of these, is recommended for improving the
general vigor of the body, for overcoming drowsiness and
indolence and, in some cases, for conquering hunger and thirst.
Here is how it is done:

Sit tailor fashion or stand relaxed, fold the tongue so that its
tip touches the upper palate, and draw air *through the mouth*
with a hissing sound. Retain the breath briefly without discomfort. Afterwards exhale through both nostrils. Another
method for exhaling is again through the mouth, with teeth
closed. Repeat three times, then rest. Neither this nor the

exercise which follows should be done out-of-doors or in a chilly room, because of the mouth-breathing involved.

Sitali is an exercise for purification of the blood. It is done as follows: Protrude the tongue slightly and fold it like a tube. Again, draw the air in through the mouth with a hissing sound, retain briefly, then exhale through both nostrils. Three times daily is enough. The Yogis say this practice "cools the system," and helps the body get rid of dyspepsia, fever, billious disorders and the effects of poison.

Bastrika relieves inflammation of the throat, clears the sinuses, cures diseases of the nose and chest and gets rid of asthma, as well as strengthening the lungs. It destroys the germs which give rise to upper respiratory disorders and gives warmth to the body in cold weather—surely a boon to those of us who live in vast, crowded urban centers with their air pollution and smog. Here is how it is practiced:

Sit tailor fashion on the floor. Start a brief rapid succession of expulsions of breath, one after another. Having done ten or twelve, draw in the breath with the deepest possible inhalation. Then suspend breathing for a few seconds, but not long enough to feel strain. Repeat three times. Like other Yoga breathing practices, this exercise must not be continued to excess.

Later on, as you learn to assume Yoga poses, or *asanas*, you may choose to do your breathing exercises while practicing one of them. This, however, is not at all necessary. What is necessary is for you to feel comfortable and relaxed when you start. This means that your clothes must be loose and never binding, that you shut out all unnecessary noise and that there be no disturbing influences in the room.

The more you increase your supply of *prana*, the greater will be your sense of well-being. In time, as you gain confidence in your ability to control *self*, you may even be able to achieve what the Yogis do—utilize *prana* for healing by consciously directing its currents to any unhealthy part of your body. What the exact process is by which this vital force acts to marshal the resources of the human body we cannot, of course, attempt to define. Nevertheless with practice even a Western student should be able to close his eyes—this in order to concentrate more perfectly—and by fixing his mind upon the sick area effect an improvement.

The advanced Yogis also frequently heal others by transmitting their own supply of *prana* through laying their hands upon the sick. By this method they give warmth, renew failing strength, relieve pain. For them even absent healing is possible, for currents of *prana* may be transmitted, like electricity, over distances and in any direction. But here a word of warning is necessary: nothing like this should ever be tried by anyone with only a slight knowledge of Yoga; in fact, experimentation in this area might prove extremely dangerous, as every *Guru* is careful to warn his disciples. For there is much too much about *prana* we do not know and it is best not to unleash magnetic forces in nature which we are so very far from understanding.

Similarly, there are dangers in any premature awakening of the Kundalini power before the student has learned full self-control and become passion-proof. If we accept the parallel between *Kundalini* and the subconscious, we can readily understand the reasons for this. Ordinarily the subconscious is buried deep under layers of civilizing disciplines, taboos and inhibitions arising out of the need of the individual to live an orderly life in a complex world among his fellow-men. But release the subconscious from all restraints, and the result may be a waking dream of the kind induced by drugs. Then, with the line between reality and fantasy blurring, the inner censor gone, who can predict what one might not be tempted to do? Illusion combined with a false sense of power can only spell danger. Fortunately, basic Yoga training carefully guards the student against foolish illusion and only a recklessly experimental attitude can possibly harm one. The sensible person, calmly following the routines we have outlined, can only benefit. At the least you will be learning to use your respiratory organs to best advantage, increasing your physical vigor. You will discover a new joy in living and a new peace of mind.

CHAPTER VI

Deep Relaxation: First Step Toward Serenity and Health

Have you ever had the experience of going to consult a doctor only to be told, after he has made his diagnosis of your physical ills: "... But your main trouble is that you are much too tense. Stop driving yourself so. Try to rest more. Try to get more sleep. *Relax!* Let down a little ..."

But if you point out to him that your nerves will not let you unwind, that when you go to bed and turn the lights out sleep will not come, that you wake in the morning as tense and weary as when finally you did drift off, the best he can do for you is to offer you a crutch. Probably a bundle of nerves himself, he will prescribe sleeping pills or tranquilizers, long walks, or a glass of warm milk at night. What he will not say, simply because he doesn't think along these lines himself, is that relaxation may be *learned* and that in learning it you begin to cope successfully with both your physical and emotional problems.

There can be no physical relaxation without the mental; no mental relaxation without the physical. This becomes self-evident as soon as you stop to think that every movement, no matter how slight, involves a nerve impulse, while every nerve impulse brings on some muscular contraction, voluntary or involuntary. If you stretch out to rest with your mind churning, for instance, you will find yourself tossing restlessly; then if you force yourself to lie still, you will feel your neck muscles tensing or realize suddenly that you are clenching your teeth.

When people say they feel like crying with sheer fatigue, they mean just that: physically, they have reached a point where the only release for their weariness is an emotional purge. Afterwards, of course, they will end up completely exhausted, for nothing eats up one's energy like letting the emotions have full play.

Most of us are spendthrifts of our energy resources. We dissipate them twenty-four hours a day. Just watch yourself and the people around you. Can you sit still, quiet and at ease, for ten or even five minutes? Or do you fidget, shift about, cross and re-cross your legs, drum with your fingers on the arm of your chair, rub your neck, bite your lips? In a roomful of people, is there even one who is without nervous habits? If so, he is a happy exception. Nor, mind you, does this apply to "busy-busy" persons alone. It is perfectly possible to spend a quiet day with nothing in the least urgent to do and still eat one's self up with tension. In fact boredom itself is an enemy in this respect. Think how many people with easy, routine jobs complain of being "dead tired" by the end of the day. And who of us hasn't said, at one time or another, "I haven't done *a thing* all day, but I'm beat."?

Unlike modern machinery, the human body was never made to cope with the stresses and strains of our civilization, with the tempo at which we live. From the moment an alarm wakes us in the morning, we begin a race with time. In order to get to work, we cover miles by car, train, bus or subway. We grab lunch in a hurry. All day long we are up against noise and pressure. And evenings are not much better, what with radio, TV, the telephone, do-it-yourself chores around the house. Moreover, the whole world around us has shrunk and is moving at an infinitely faster pace in this atomic age when planes and rockets have linked the continents and space travel is the reality of tomorrow.

At the same time an alarming barrage of illnesses termed psychogenic and psychosomatic—that is, originating in the psyche or mind—is bedevilling twentieth-century man. To mention only a few, ulcers and colitis—notorious disturbances of nervous origin and both relatively rare a generation ago—are becoming more and more frequent. Heart disease is taking an ever heavier toll of relatively young people, especially those working at high-power jobs and living on their nerves.

This is by no means coincidental. There is a direct correlation between the ills of our world and the ills of our body. Even those of us who have little taste for living at breakneck speed cannot completely escape the effects of the speed-up, for no man is an island and the bell tolls for all of us. So we fall heir to the minor ills of the age—nervous fatigue, nervous indigestion, sleep that leaves us unrefreshed, strain, irritability—all of them fertile soil for trouble later on. Yet the doctors, who understand so well where all this may lead and who can explain *in principle* the dangers of tensions, can suggest no better remedy than for you to "change your ways." How you are to accomplish this is, to use the popular phrase, your own problem.

Before we go on to a discussion of the actual techniques of Deep Relaxation, let us consider for a moment what relaxation is not. In the first place, it is *not* play. Nor is it a change of pace or of occupation. Play and change are fine, of course. They do help, they are a step in the right direction. But they are not the real thing.

Thus the tired businessman out for a day of golf, the home gardener, the knitter, the Sunday painter, are all people who indulge in pleasant hobbies in order to get away from other routines, but they are merely substituting one form of activity for another. The same holds true for the avid reader, the Hi-Fi enthusiast, the TV fan. Each finds a degree of respite in doing what he enjoys, but each remains occupied. The mind keeps ticking away, the muscles remain at work. Even listening to music with the eyes closed requires a certain expenditure of energy! Very definitely, *recreation* cannot be considered true, complete relaxation.

Quite possibly one reason why we Americans find it so difficult to take time out for "doing nothing" is that for generations it has been drilled into us that idleness was a cardinal sin. Our Puritan ancestors were firmly convinced that not a moment of the waking day must be wasted, for didn't the devil provide work for idle fingers? So if you have a hangover of childhood guilt on the subject, here is an idea worth exploring: Consider how much more alert you become after a few minutes of true relaxation—how much more you are able to accomplish in your working time *as well as* your playtime, if you bring to it a free, clear, deeply rested mind. If you learn to rest, you can work that much better.

Once in a rare while someone does stumble on the secret of relaxation without being taught. Napoleon is said to have been a master of it; he could actually sleep on horseback, with his eyes open—which simply meant he could withdraw from his surroundings and relax at will. Five or ten minutes later he could rouse himself, as refreshed as if he had slept for hours. Consequently he was tireless and got along on no more than four or five hours' actual sleep a night.

Franklin D. Roosevelt had that same capacity. Churchill had it. During the most trying war years, when there was no time for rest, both of these men would switch off their energy at its source, give it a chance to replenish itself—and the whole world became the gainer. Most of us are not so skillful. Animals, on the other hand, possess the secret of complete relaxation from the day they are born. Not even contact with civilized man causes them to lose it.

As we have already mentioned, the Yogis, observing this difference between man and beast, began thousands of years ago to learn from it. They related the animal's total relaxation in sleep, in rest and especially during hibernation—that trance-like sleep or state of suspended animation which lasts the winter and makes it unnecessary to forage for food while none is available—to a capacity for retaining youth and vigor. Wisely they based a great many of their own practices on what they learned.

In fact, most of the Yoga exercises and postures, or *asanas*, derive from study of animal life. Many are even named for animals—the *Cobra* pose, the *Lion* pose. As for Deep Relaxation, during which you will learn to "let go" as many muscles as possible and as many thoughts as possible so that both brain and body may rest to the very core of your being, this is done in the most ancient of all basic Yoga postures, *Savasana*, which in Sanskrit means the "Death Pose." Fortunately, however, *Savasana* does not relate to death; only to hibernation, which has to do with prolongation of life.

As you embark on your first Deep Relaxation exercises, try to bear in mind that the object of what you will do is to quiet your nerves and rest your body by ridding yourself of all conscious tension and contraction. Perhaps you want to overcome that lethal habit, worry. Perhaps your problem is lack of vitality, fatigue, or poor concentration. You may be wearing yourself out by remaining constantly on the go and must learn to give yourself moments of respite; or you may need the respite because you never seem to gather enough energy for getting started on whatever it is you mean to do.

Tension is your big problem. Tension is the enemy of achievement. "Easy does it" is not a meaningless saying—it is a basic truth whose meaning we too often ignore. Whether you happen to be an artist hoping to paint a masterpiece, an athlete on the way toward a championship or just an average human being who would like to live to the full potential of his capacity, you are much more likely to achieve your goal if you don't try too hard.

True, to learn to relax completely takes practice, and cannot be mastered in one easy lesson. But you will certainly learn how if you are willing to try. Moreover, from the very beginning, even while you are still unable to let go completely, you will begin to feel the benefits of what you are doing. And this, in turn, will make for more success: you will have started a benign instead of a vicious circle. Soon your nervous system will become like a complicated network of highly charged electric wires with the current turned off: no hum, no sparks, no vibrations, while the batteries that are the mainspring of energy recharge themselves.

We have mentioned that there are over four hundred muscles on each side of the human body—no fewer than twenty in the forearm alone. Most of the time we are not even conscious of using half of them. Moreover, we use them in groups and many of the small ones are beyond the range of our conscious feeling. Certainly we do not tense them consciously, nor would we know how to let go of them consciously.

And now for the actual techniques of Deep Relaxation, the step-by-step approaches:

Since routine is always helpful in acquiring good habits, do try, whenever possible, to do your relaxing exercises at approximately the same time each day. Early morning or late evening, for instance, might be a desirable time for several reasons: Early morning relaxation helps insure a good, serene day; a late evening period is a good preamble to a restful night's sleep. On the other hand, you might be one of those people who need to replenish their energies at the end of the working day. In deciding what is best for you, your guide should always be your own ease and comfort. Any sense of "must," of pressure, should be avoided.

Until you have become so adept at relaxing that you can, like Napoleon, shut out the world around you at any time and any place, your period of relaxation should be taken away from other people, in a room where you are alone, with the door closed. You will need quiet so as not to be distracted. If you are a city dweller you doubtless cannot avoid a certain amount of traffic noise, but try to control what sounds you can, since conversation, the radio, the ticking of a clock can be most distracting. Keep disturbance at a minimum.

Your clothes should be comfortable, too. In fact, the less you have on the better: Make certain you are not annoyed by a tight belt, a stiff collar, a girdle, a brassiere. Anything that might make you unduly conscious of being physically confined should be avoided. On the other hand you must not feel cold. Be sure there are no drafts in the room—it is impossible to relax properly while chilly.

The best possible position for Deep Relaxation, as you may have guessed, is the *Savasana*, the Death Pose. And the best place is the floor. Lie flat on your back, using a rug or folded blanket to protect yourself from the cold boards. If for some reason it is impossible for you to use the floor, then choose a hard bed, preferably one with a bed board. A soft bed will never be completely satisfactory, for as it sags under your weight, certain muscles will inevitably tense up. Moreover, a soft bed might lull you to sleep, and sleep is *not* what you are after at the moment.

You will probably not feel entirely comfortable when you first try lying like this: The floor will feel too hard, you will find yourself tempted to shift positions. But this you must not do, for in order to relax muscle by muscle it is important to lie quite still. Just remember that every body movement, every shift, however slight, means a tensing of one or another group of muscles. To avoid this, make sure that you are lying comfortably, with your weight fairly evenly distributed.

Once settled, take a few deep breaths from the diaphragm, as you have learned in the previous chapter; then allow yourself to breathe normally again. The next step is to get acquainted with the *feel* of your muscles so that you may better control them. Pretend you have swallowed a tracer substance, and that your muscles are channels through which you are watching it flow.

Now send an order along one of these channels. Move an arm, stretch a leg. Stretch hard, making all the muscles along the way contract—and study what is happening. You will feel muscles quite far removed from the area with which you are experimenting contract in sympathy. If you clench your fist, for instance, you will feel contractions all the way up your arm and into your shoulder. If you flex your toes, ripples of movement will tense the muscles of your thigh.

Now hold the stretch a moment, while you trace your sensations in detail. Memorize them: next time you give your arm an order, you will be able to check whether or not it is being followed. And now let go. Repeat the process limb by limb, until you have a nodding acquaintance with the various groups of muscles through your body.

Now start the stretching all over again, but this time in slow motion. Build the stretch up, slowly, like a cat arching its back. In the meantime let the imaginary tracer substance show you, as clearly as possible, every muscle you have put into play. Observe and note your sensations for future reference. Hold the pose until you are thoroughly aware of what is happening. Then, once more in slow motion, let go.

It is this letting-go process that is the actual mechanism of true relaxation. Think of yourself as a puppet without any strings to hold it up any longer—could anything be more limp? That is the stage you are trying to reach—relaxation so complete that you lose all feeling of alertness. This is your goal.

As has already been said, you are not likely to achieve such a state on your first attempt, nor even the second. Most people make better progress in the end if, instead of trying to relax the entire body at once, they concentrate on some one part. Start, for instance, with an arm. Pretend it is a length of old rope. Let the shoulder fall inert, heavy, on the floor. Let the rest follow, all the way down the arm, until inertia has traveled through elbow, forearm, wrist and palm and the fingers feel like the rope's limp, raveled ends.

After you have done this several times, start concentrating on your legs. See if you can make your neck and spine feel like so much jelly. After a while relaxation will become a habit and you will no longer need to think of specific areas; you will have learned to relax the entire body as a coordinated unit. When that time comes, you will have learned to rest as you have never rested in your whole life; you will discover a totally new sense of well-being, alertness and serenity.

Once you have mastered the basic approaches, you will start developing a definite sequence, a routine for Deep Relaxation. It has been found that the most effective way to relax is to begin at the top and work down: Relax the head first—let go the face muscles, the jaw muscles, the eyeballs, the lips, the tongue. Pretend a slow current of water is flowing through you, cleansing your body of tension. Let it flow through your neck, down the shoulders into the arms, down the chest into the abdomen, down your spine and through your buttocks, your thighs, knees, calves and into your legs, trickling out finally through your toes. In the end, your body will have no more tone than the body of a rag doll.

But even after you have grown quite adept at doing all this, you will discover from time to time that muscle-groups are tensing up once more or that you simply have passed some by. They must be relaxed again, of course. Moreover, after you first feel yourself relax all over, you will find you are capable of repeating the process on a deeper level—it is as though you had walked into a very quiet, deep forest, rested awhile, then walked on to where the trees are denser still and the silence deeper. In the end you will be on the very verge of drowsiness, of total inertia, your mind virtually at a standstill. When you have reached that stage, you will be resting in every cell of your body.

Students usually ask how long the daily period of Deep Relaxation should last. There can be no hard and fast rule for this, especially since time-span varies with quality: the deeper the degree of relaxation, the more benefit you derive from it and the less time you need. At first plan on fifteen minutes or even half an hour a day. Later on you will find even a ten-minute period beneficial. You will also discover that a few minutes' Deep Relaxation just as you are *on the verge* of getting tired but are not yet headed toward exhaustion is a wise rule. It will revitalize you, giving you second wind, whenever during the day your energies are flagging.

As for the correct time at which to terminate the exercise—your own body will tell you when it is ready to get back into action. Remember, however, never to get up hastily or jerkily, or you will be undoing the benefits of the *asana*. The proper way to end a period of Deep Relaxation is to work your way down the muscles of the body one final time; but now you must reverse the process: Instead of relaxing, restore tone control to each muscle group. Contract or stretch it, then go on to another group until you have tensed them all. Conclude with one final, luxurious, cat-like stretch.

Much later, after these techniques have become automatic and you have mastered greater control of your mental processes as well, you will be able to relax with people around you. You will be able to practice relaxation sitting down. And while this latter routine can never completely take the place of Deep Relaxation in the Death Pose, since no matter how comfortably seated you may be the very act of sitting up involves a certain amount of tension of spine and neck muscles, it still is an invaluable adjunct to resting. Once you have learned to divorce yourself at will from the world of action around you, merely sitting still a few moments with the eyes closed and the mind more or less a blank can be a wonderful weapon against nervous fatigue and exhaustion.

A great many persons make the mistake of assuming that if a period of relaxation is good, an equivalent amount of time spent napping must be better. As a matter of scientific fact, the opposite is true. Sleep, whether at night or during catnaps is a fine way to rest the body. But it is the rare man or woman who relaxes thoroughly in sleep. Most of us toss and turn, and so continue tensing our muscles all night long.

Deep Relaxation, on the other hand, since it is based on immobility, ensures total rest. It is a conscious, willed process, controlled by the mind which, in turn, relaxes thoroughly as the muscles begin to sag. In sleep we are likely to be fatigued by the dreams which plague our subconscious, for we all do dream, whether or not we remember our dreams. But resting while awake, after having emptied the mind of worrisome thoughts, means reaching a state of true mental repose. Thus a half hour of deepest relaxation can refresh an exhausted person as hours of fitful sleep never would.

This is how the Yogis sum it all up:

Peaceful repose is derived in two ways: from *Ananda*, the bliss of sleep, which comes to everyone in a healthy state; and from *Samadhi*, or relaxation. And the difference between the two is that in the former there is a veil of ignorance, whereas in the latter there is no veil: therefore, *Samadhi* is superior to *Ananda*.

Moreover, to master Deep Relaxation is the first step toward the more advanced stages of Yoga practice, Concentration and Meditation. And the difference between them is that in Relaxation the mind is made passive and you allow thoughts to flow in;

whereas in Concentration and Meditation the mind is made to fix upon some central point and shut out all thoughts but the one upon which the attention is turned by choice. However, these higher stages cannot be achieved without first passing through the first one.

Deep Relaxation, then, is the first step toward serenity of spirit and health of body.

CHAPTER VII

Deep Contraction: The Way to Vitality and Strength

After every action there must be a reaction. Now that you have the key to complete deep relaxation, the next step is to learn *Deep Contraction*. The two together will enable you to better utilize the full potential of your body and mind and gear them to working for you. Think of this as a preliminary mobilization of all your resources for approaching the more complex physical and mental routines you will be trying later on.

We already know that Yoga relaxation has nothing in common with relaxation as it is understood by most people in the Western world who equate it with rest, recreation or play. Similarly, Deep Contraction has nothing to do with various methods of "toning up" or "keeping fit" with which we are familiar. Nothing can be further from Yoga practice than subjecting the body to physical drills. Deep knee bends, push-ups, weight-lifting—all the routines generally associated with physical culture—are the very antithesis of what Yoga tries to accomplish. For while such drills are fine for the young and the athletic, they encourage muscle tension in the average person for whom tension is usually already a problem. Realistically, too, they require more daily effort than anyone but an athlete is likely to be willing to make. But most importantly they tend to dissociate body from mind, while the Yoga approach is always to consider the human whole, treating it as indivisible.

The greatest of modern theatrical directors, Constantin Stanislavski, to whose techniques actors throughout the world refer with bated breath simply as "The Method," advised his students to learn from animals how to first relax, then "wind up" for perfect body control. "Watch the tiger," he wrote in *An Actor Prepares*, "watch his domesticated counterpart, the cat. See how completely they let go of every muscle, becoming a dead weight in sleep or relaxation. Then watch them as they wake: they stretch, yawn, slowly get to their feet and arch their back, changing from limp rag to coiled spring with no apparent effort."

What Stanislavski wanted to demonstrate was the tremendous economy of energy and movement which gives the feline its peculiar grace and power. Thus he was able to teach his students how to move, tireless, through taxing emotional roles; how to breathe so that their voices projected, without ever straining, to every corner of a great hall even if used in a whisper. It is not surprising to learn that he had studied the methods of Hatha Yoga.

Most of us will never be called upon to play Hamlet or King Lear eight times a week, to sing in Grand Opera or to go barnstorming through the country for a presidential candidate. Nor will we attempt to chalk up Olympic Games records. But we have it within our reach to learn quickly and all but effortlessly a kind of body control that even the fine athlete doesn't always possess since he too, unless he is either naturally lucky or has learned the secret of alternate relaxation and contraction, is likely to be laboring under much unnecessary tension.

Animals, unlike man, know instinctively how to keep fit. Yet their "secret" is simplicity itself. It consists merely of indulging in the most stimulating physical exercise there is— natural, spontaneous body movements. Let us go back for a moment to the awakening tiger-kitten: The yawn and big stretch are nothing more nor less than passive forms of deep muscular contraction after a period of Deep Relaxation—contraction that reaches into every muscle group from head to toes. Then, after he has awakened his sinews in this pleasant and satisfying manner, the kitten suddenly leaps after a speck of dust. He has gone from passive into active contraction. The motion, you will notice, is effortless. An animal never tries to prove anything; he moves for the sheer pleasure of being in motion.

One of the reasons why Western physical culture is unsatisfactory except for the young and the athletic is that in addition to tiring and over-exerting already weary hearts and arteries it tends to develop the body unevenly. It concentrates on certain muscle groups while never involving others, so that body imbalance is likely to follow. Over-zealous athletes often become muscle-bound. This means ugly bulges, stiffness and an inability to let go, which sometimes has to be treated by massage. Middle-aged men and women who once were athletes, on the other hand, tend to suffer from flabbiness—the result of formerly over-developed muscles now gone to seed. This in turn invites stiffness, rheumatism, neuritis and rheumatoid arthritis. But when muscles stretch during Deep Contraction, a lubricant called synovial fluid is immediately secreted, helping disperse the waste matter which causes stiffness at the joints. At the same time lymph flows more freely, nourishing and stimulating body cells. Blood circulation is improved, of course, because you are breathing properly.

Expensive slenderizing salons are filled with persons of both sexes who are looking for their lost youth and their lost figures, letting themselves be pummelled and shaken up on massage tables and in electrical contraptions. How much wiser and pleasanter for them if they turned to the *natural* method of Deep Contraction. Not only would the results be more far-reaching, but far longer-lasting as well.

As a matter of fact, Deep Contraction can form a bridge to ease you, all but effortlessly, into the more difficult phase of learning the Yoga postures on which the Deep Contraction method itself is based. Once you have grasped the underlying principle and formed the habit of regular routine, your body will quickly begin to grow limber, your muscles and tendons elastic, so that when you are ready to try your first *asana*, you will not find it too difficult. In the meantime your muscle tone will be improving, stiffness disappearing and your figure getting back to its youthful *optimum*, all because Deep Contraction, along with Dynamic Breathing, tones the body, stimulates circulation and causes waste to be carried away and deposits of fat and calcium to be utilized instead of remaining a dead weight.

As we have just pointed out, Deep Contraction routines are based on the most important of Yoga *asanas*. Like these asanas, all Deep Contraction is nothing more nor less than a prolongation of natural, instinctive stretches carried to the point where a person's whole mood and physique become involved. Bear in mind that you will not be expected to try poses which require endless application, for these are wholly unsuited to our Occidental way of life. Instead, you will be given a few of the simple, albeit important poses which may be learned in easy stages by any ordinary Westerner, even one used to sedentary living. Nor should age be a barrier, or lack of stamina. All you are asked to keep in mind is that you must not over-exert yourself.

At the very first, begin by practicing stretches of your own devising. Do whatever is comfortable and natural, only make sure that you do your stretching three different ways: lying flat on your back, sitting down, and standing upright. You might begin, as suggested in Chapter III, by taking a good stretch when you wake in the morning, taking a tip from our friend the tiger-cat. Rather than jump out of bed, take a minute or two to yawn, stretch your legs, feet and toes as far as possible, stretch your arms high above your head, stretch your neck, your chest, your waist and your back. Above all, let every movement be natural, unhurried, fluid. During each stretch try to contract as many muscles as you can consciously trace. Then hold the stretch for as long as a minute, building up tension gradually. Then, just as gradually, let down again. Remember never to move jerkily, since this negates the benefits of the exercise.

Repeat the same kind of stretching several times during the day, at least once while sitting in a chair and once while you are standing. Try to allot five minutes in all to these three routines. Remember to pay especial attention to the waist and the back, for in that way you will be benefiting two vital areas —the spinal column and the abdominal cavity; in other words, you will be toning the main trunk-line of your nervous system and the internal organs concerned with digestion and elimination.

At the end of a few days, when you have begun to feel completely natural in your stretching routines, you can go on to the next step, which is to do your Deep Contraction exercises directly following the relaxation period. Remember, during Deep Relaxation you have been lying flat on the floor on your back, eyes closed, arms along your sides, in the *Savasana* or Death Pose. Now, as you rouse yourself, start lifting both legs from the hips, toes pointed and knees held straight. Do this *slowly* being careful to keep the rest of your body, neck and head down on the floor. Lift as high as you can, preferably until your legs are at a right angle with your body, always being careful to notice the various contractions that begin with the feet, extend up the calf, through the thighs and into the abdominal region. Hold this stretch for as long as possible without feeling strain. Then, slowly and gently, lower the feet to the floor in one smooth movement. Then rest. You probably don't know it, but you have just completed the first step toward learning two extremely important *asanas*—the *Sarvangasana*, or Cradle Posture, and the *Halasana*, or Plough, whose benefits will be discussed elsewhere.

Next sit up and try grasping your toes or ankles with your hands, bending the trunk and keeping the legs stretched out. Continue to bend as far forward as possible, holding this position for a few moments before loosening your grip and slowly sitting up once more. Do not worry if at first you are unable to grasp your feet. You will gradually grow more limber as you continue exercising a little every day. The main thing to keep in mind is that *you are doing the best you can*—and not to overtax yourself. Remember, too, to avoid jerky motions: the stretch should be natural. Again you have just completed the first step in a Yoga posture which has special value in strengthening the abdomen and spine, the *Paschimottanasana* (see Chapter XI).

Now lie flat on your stomach, keeping your legs straight out. Place your hands on the floor in line with the shoulders. Try to lift yourself by pressing down on the hands. At first this may seem hard, but after a week or so you will be able to lift your whole body from the hips up—and you will have performed the first part of the *Bhujangasana*, or Snake Posture (See Chapter XI), which is excellent for the spine.

Your last stretch is to be done standing. Stand with the feet slightly apart, knees slightly bent. Place the hands on the thighs. Take a deep breath, exhale, then expel the breath sharply. Now try to draw the abdomen in and up, raising the diaphragm as high as possible. Hold this position a moment, then relax. You have completed the first step toward the *Uddiyana Bandha* (see Chapter XI), an *asana* which massages the colon, the large and small intestines, and starts peristaltic action, generally doing away with any tendency to constipation by envigorating the nerves which control intestinal movements. Moreover, muscles which ordinarily are beyond our voluntary control are involved here. This is an exercise which also helps a fallen stomach, intestines or uterus. It should, of course, always be done on an empty stomach.

Ideally, when you try this final routine the stomach should be sucked in so deep that it practically disappears. But the beginning student is hardly likely to achieve anything like such an effect, for the average person's neglected abdominal muscles are apt to be weak and unresponsive. However, here again you are not striving for perfection. This, like the previous routines, should be in the nature of a glorified stretch. Do not ask too much of yourself. Be content to make haste slowly.

As to timing—each of the above four exercises should take about a minute so that, with rests in between, you should allow five minutes for the lot. Get in the habit of doing them immediately after your Deep Relaxation period, either before breakfast or the last thing at night. If neither time is feasible, find some other convenient break during the day. But always be sure to wear loose, comfortable clothing and to allow at least two and preferably three hours to elapse after a meal before you begin.

In order to get the full benefit of both the relaxation and the contraction, remember that your mental attitude is of the greatest importance. It is useless to go through the motions of exercising unless you are prepared to focus your entire attention on what you are doing. Just as, during relaxation, you must empty your mind of all distracting influences, so during the stretches you must teach yourself to dwell on their performance only, to study each action and its effects on your body, allowing yourself to relish the sensations you are experiencing. Only if you are thoroughly aware of the good you are doing yourself will the benefit of the routines stay with you. On the other hand, if you do follow the routine faithfully you will begin to acquire greater limberness and to experience both physical and mental well-being within one short week. You will sleep better, have greater vitality and your nerves will be your friends instead of traitors.

Even if you never do progress to the more complicated forms of Yoga exercise and content yourself merely with the first three steps—Dynamic Breathing, Deep Relaxation and Contraction—the benefits you will derive will astonish you. This is so because, from the very first, the emphasis here is not on building up one or another part of your body, not on one or another "angle," but on the whole being. For at all stages Yoga aims at creating a balanced mental-physical combination of improvement and growth. In the process, especially during Deep Contraction exercises, certain muscle groups and skin areas are brought into play which during ordinary physical drills remain unaffected. The skin, specially, is stretched and pulled and stimulated so that it gets the benefit of thorough cleansing and flushing. When you consider that a piece of skin the size of a postage stamp contains some three million separate cells, a yard of blood vessels, four yards of nerves and twenty-five nerve endings, not to mention hundreds of sweat and oil glands, and when you realize that ordinary exercise doesn't

begin to wake up all this complex organism, you really understand why the Yoga approach is like no other—why it seems
to show the way to the Fountain of Youth. Healthy, well-
nourished skin will not sag nor grow sallow nor wrinkle. And
even tired skin, after a little systematic Yoga stimulation, can
once more acquire the firmness and glow it once had. And
this is only a secondary benefit!

The complex of processes which constitutes Deep Contraction has one final, most important aspect which so far we
only mentioned in passing while discussing mental attitude.
We have pointed out that it would be quite useless, not to say
impossible, to practice true Deep Contraction while thinking
of something else. This orientation inward, which becomes a
must, is the first step toward a further, deeper development
of your Self according to Yoga principles. For once you have
learned Deep Contraction and have practiced it for a while,
you are ready to go on to something still more important,
something essential not only to the welfare of your body but
of your entire being: You are ready to learn Concentration.

CHAPTER VIII

Concentration: Key to Mastery
Of the Mind and the Emotions

The mind should be the willing servant of the Self. But it is only the very rare man or woman who possesses sufficient natural self-discipline for achieving this. In the case of most of us, the mind is either helpless slave or tyrannical master. Lacking proper orientation, we permit the impact of the world around us forever to impinge on us. Some of us let ourselves be buffeted by emotional storms or are forever being distracted by external stimuli, with the result that single-minded pursuit of what is truly important to us is all but impossible. Others tend to veer to the other extreme; in an effort to set up defenses against external or emotional distraction we become creatures of the mind exclusively, denying natural impulses, rigid and driven in outlook. Thus in one way or another our very efforts at self-discipline defeat us, consuming energy which might more happily be put to constructive, creative use.

These are failings of human nature as old as human nature itself. The Yogis, wisely aware of them, long ago devised a method for dealing with the problem. Just as their physical training teaches the student to get the most out of the potential of his body, so their mental disciplines are a key to teaching the individual how to function at one hundred percent capacity on the emotional and intellectual level.

This key may be called Deep Concentration.

Relaxation and Contraction, which you have learned in the two previous chapters, in addition to being necessary and highly beneficial in themselves, may also be regarded as pre-liminary steps to Concentration. Although both require a certain amount of mental discipline, they are primarily physical routines. Now, however, you are on a truly different plane. Yet it is always well to bear in mind that there is no arbitrary division between the two, since body and mind are indivisible in all their interrelationships.

Yoga teaches that in order to control the mind one must first learn to empty it of useless baggage. Most of us live our lives out with our thoughts a needless clutter, the essential and the non-essential crowded together helter-skelter. Civilized man's mind, like his body, tends to be overloaded. But just as our bodies can grow firmer and lighter if we follow proper Yoga breathing and exercise routines, so we can learn to travel light mentally, discarding whatever doesn't properly belong, allowing instead plenty of space and light for the essentials to thrive in.

Since obviously there can be no such thing as concentration in a mental vacuum, one must always concentrate *on some-thing*. That is the first lesson to be learned. You must focus your attention on some image or object while determinedly shutting out everything else. This is not nearly so easy as it sounds—try thinking of one single thing for a period of thirty seconds, and see what happens! Left to itself the mind tends to flit from subject to subject, free-associating at a great rate. Keeping it from these gymnastics is the very essence of the problem.

During Deep Relaxation, you will remember, it was important to discipline your thinking in order to keep your mind from stimulating and tensing your muscles. In Deep Concentration, the same initial effort is called for, but with a difference: whereas in relaxation the mind must be made as nearly blank as possible, in Deep Concentration it is made to dwell closely, steadily, on one thing and one alone.

The various schools of Yoga teach various beginnings, but they almost invariably start by suggesting concentration on some part of the body. Thus *Raja Yoga* advises focusing on

Trikute, the seat of the mind, which is said to be either the top of the head or the space between the eyes. Other schools recommend focusing on the tip of the nose, the navel or the *Muladhara Chakra* (see pages 58–59), the space directly below the last vertebra at the base of the spine. An excellent way to begin practice is to seat yourself in a comfortable position— tailor fashion on the floor is recommended, but not absolutely necessary—and look steadily at an object directly in your line of vision. Next shut your eyes and try to visualize the object clearly in the space between your eyebrows. You will find in very short order that the picture fades from your mental vision. When this happens open your eyes, refresh the impression, and try again. At first you may have considerable difficulty in keeping the mental picture clear. Not only will it tend to fade, but you will be tempted to substitute other pictures in quick succession. External stimuli—sounds, sensations, memories—will be another constant distraction. You will have to be quite stern with yourself. But the effort will be well worth making, for if you persist you will find it progressively easier to shut out unbidden interruptions and with practice you will be able to ignore them completely for as long as it suits you.

The Hindus, whose goals are so vastly different from ours, strive through concentration and meditation for the state of Samadhi, or super-consciousness, which as you already know may best be described as that state where the Self ceases to exist and becomes absorbed in the Absolute. This is a practice definitely not to be attempted without the guidance of a *Guru*, for such deep and intense concentration may result in a sort of spiritual intoxication nothing short of an unbalanced state of mind. Useless, excessive dreaminess may also result from over-doing the exercise. For the Westerner the goal of Deep Con-centration is a far more practical one; you can learn so to harness and discipline your thinking that you will soon be bringing increased efficiency to your daily tasks, be they problems on your job, in your household, or in some creative field of your choosing.

It goes without saying that to concentrate properly one must keep serene, which means emptying the mind of irritation, worry and distraction, not permitting any of these emotions to take hold and interfere. This too becomes a matter of practice. At first, as you try concentrating on the object of your choice, you will find the immediate preoccupations of daily living crowding you, hammering for admittance. The way to deal with them is deliberately to shut them out. Learn to watch your thoughts as though you were an interested spectator but do not permit yourself to identify with them. Then, when you see them begin to wander, shepherd them back where you want them. Dull and uninspired as this will seem at first—for day-dreaming and wool-gathering are a more attractive pastime than concentrating on, say the flame of a candle—the practice will soon yield rewards. It will surprise you how quickly a little mechanical exercise will enable you so to discipline your mind that when you are called on to focus on something important, something vital, it will no longer be tempted to wander at all.

Many people make the mistake of assuming that concentration is a grim, tension-provoking business. They frown, bite a pencil, chew lips and nails in an outward show of effort. But all they succeed in doing is to increase their own restlessness, tiring themselves out to no purpose. They keep their five senses relentlessly at play, pulling in all directions instead of working together, harmoniously. That this is a profligate waste of energy both muscular and emotional, is self-evident. With Deep Concentration such frittering-away of one's resources can be avoided. You might sum it up this way: Just as at first you had to learn to concentrate in order to relax, so now you must learn to relax in order to concentrate to good advantage.

As with other Yoga routines, it is important to make a habit of practicing Deep Concentration at regular intervals, setting aside at least one regular period for it each day. You might, for instance, plan to do it immediately after the relaxation and contraction exercises in the morning, before you start on your day's chores. Late afternoon, or at night before retiring are other good times. Each has its own advantages: the morning time helps you start the day with a clear head, an afternoon period refreshes you for the evening ahead. Concentration the last thing at night offers certain very special rewards, however. As you learn greater and greater mind control, you will find that you can train yourself to project your thinking into your sleep, or toward the tasks and problems of the following day. Actually what happens is that while you sleep your innermost mind continues to function and the following morning you are likely to wake with solutions to puzzling questions clear in your mind and with an added awareness of how to go about doing what should be done.

This approach, which the Yogis worked out generations ago and which a few intuitive people are forever rediscovering for themselves is today recognized by psychiatrists as a mental process on the subconscious level. As Sigmund Freud pointed out not so very many years back for the benefit of the Western world, civilized man has buried this subconscious so deep under layers of repression and doubt that often it works against him rather than for him. The Yoga method, through Deep Concentration, helps us make friends with it once more.

Valuable as concentration directly before sleep can be to you, it is a mistake to try practicing it if, by the time you are ready for bed, you have reached a stage of mental fatigue. But if you are determined to go through with it just the same, a period of relaxation should precede it. In such a case follow the classic method: lie flat on your back, close your eyes and consciously relax each set of muscles in turn, starting with the head, neck and shoulders, going down the arms, the torso, the thighs and knees and legs, all the way into your toes. Make your mind a blank. Soon you will feel sufficiently refreshed to proceed to the mental exercises. This approach will also contribute to deep, healthful sleep.

Tired or not, never make the mistake of trying to achieve your goal of concentration by *forcing* unwelcome or irrelevant thoughts sternly out of your head. Instead, deliberately substitute those thoughts which are acceptable. For example, if you are concentrating on the flame of a candle and your mind wanders away to the picture of an ordinary light bulb, and from there to the lamp on your desk and the work piled up beside it, do not shudder away from the sight—ignore it. Focus your mind's eye on the candle flame once more. Continue doing this until your thoughts, accepting your bidding, flow as you would have them flow. But be sure again, to do this without identifying with the thoughts themselves: pretend to be the outsider looking on, as though what is going on inside your mind were an action on a stage. Always bear in mind the difference between you, the thinker, and the object of your thoughts.

This trick of looking inside yourself is the initial step toward becoming truly 'self'-conscious—conscious of the Self, that is; once you learn to separate the Self from its environment you will experience a sense of freedom and augmented strength, for then the environment, the things that are happening, the people around you, will cease to dominate your consciousness. Gone will be the need to yield to every outside demand. You will begin to cultivate the kind of detachment which will make it possible for you to be in true control of your own mind.

Many years ago Yoga was defined as "the complete mastery of the mind and emotions." You can readily see how great a part concentration plays in reaching this mastery. For as man thinks, so he is. Thus, although we are always being told that it is impossible to change human nature, you, the individual, can indeed change yourself to a very great extent by determining what your thoughts will be. For the mind is wonderfully flexible and will respond to cultivation as fertile soil responds to it. Think peace, and gradually your entire outlook becomes one of serenity and inner calm. Empty your mind of anger, of resentment against your fellow-beings, substitute an attitude of live-and-let-live, and you will be rewarded by a sense of tolerance that will make living with others infinitely easier. Refuse to be ruffled by the thousand-and-one phenomena that yesterday distracted you from your chosen course, and a deep and genuine feeling of equanimity will soon make it easier for you to live with yourself and, of course, with others.

The Yogis go much further. They claim that the mind of each of us influences the minds of others by means of currents we set up. Therefore, they say, harsh and hostile thoughts spread harm and may actually *do harm* to those who come in contact with us while on the contrary calm and kindness contribute to their well-being. Be that as it may, we do know— and both medical men and psychologists are the first to agree with this—a hostile, negative attitude is invariably destructive both to ourselves and to our relationships with others. The only constructive approach is the positive one. Through practice of Yoga it is possible to achieve such an attitude without having recourse to such long, arduous processes of emotional re-education as people are given on the psychiatrist's couch. It would be the height of folly not to profit by what is at hand.

For the ordinary person, there is, of course, no such thing as complete detachment. The highly-trained Yogi on the other hand is able so completely to detach himself from the world around him that he achieves startling results. For instance, it is basically through intense concentration—through his single-minded refusal to permit any outside manifestation whatsoever to disrupt it—that the Indian fakir learns so completely to control his body as to perform the feats for which fakirs are famous. Suspending breath for days at a time, halting the beating of the heart, sitting on a bed of nails without any seeming ill-effects—all these are the more spectacular results of complete, intensive concentration combined with the exercise of highly-developed will power. We in the West aren't interested in such accomplishments. If the fakirs' feats are mentioned here at all, it is only to demonstrate to what extraordinary lengths it is possible to triumph over normal human limitations. Our immediate interest is to learn to benefit from concentration in practical ways.

In the chapter on Meditation which follows we shall look at the further benefits derived from that deepening of self-knowledge to which correct thinking inevitably leads. But the beginnings of this self-knowledge are right here. For as your mind becomes impervious to disturbance from within as well as without, as you grow less vulnerable, so to speak, the thousand tensions set up by ever-present emotional conflicts gradually disappear. As your thinking becomes less chaotic, as you learn to stay with an idea, pleasant or unpleasant, until you have really given yourself a chance to examine it closely, not only do you become able to face your real self honestly but, whatever facts you discover about yourself, you can face them with equanimity. Next, the need which all of us have to keep up a façade gradually vanishes. This in turn helps us live each day with a more economic outlay of emotional resources.

And now for a few simple exercises to teach you to harness the powerhouse of your mind. The goals are simple at first. Like all Yoga exercises they should be done without the threat of interruptions, while you are alone in a room. Your clothes and your position should be comfortable. Everything should contribute to an initial attitude of relaxation.

Intense concentration can improve memory, since lack of it is largely a matter of inability to focus on anything long enough or with sufficient interest, for it to make a lasting impression. A simple exercise which does not even require the traditional Yoga pose is to select a few cards out of a pack, lay them face down in front of you, then jot down the value and suit of each. With practice you will be able to increase the number of cards you are able to remember at one time until finally you will accurately recall the entire pack in the order in which you put them down.

An auxiliary exercise which may be practiced profitably at odd moments is to make yourself consciously aware of what you see as you walk down a street or enter a room. Rather than proceed in your usual state of semi-consciousness, try making a point of assimilating as many impressions as possible. After-wards try just as systematically to recall as many as you can after you have reached your destination. This, by the way, is a good preliminary to the more formal, and more difficult, practice of sitting with the eyes closed and systematically making yourself remember everything you did during the previous day. You will probably be amazed at first at how many details actually escape you. In time, however, you will learn to marshal your thoughts until yesterday's events pass clearly in review before your mind's eye like a series of motion picture stills projected on a screen. Remember, do not be tempted to pick and choose, shrugging off certain memories as too trivial and inconsequential to merit notice. They doubtless are, in themselves, but it isn't their intrinsic importance with which you are concerned for the moment. Remember you are now engaged in a training process intended to develop your ability to control not just your memory, but those thoughts which are important to you.

A final exercise in concentration, and the most difficult of all for reasons which are self-evident, is to spend a few minutes nightly reviewing the day's happenings and scrutinizing your own behaviour directly before you fall asleep. The difficulty here is not that your tired mind will be tempted to wander. A far more serious stumbling block is the simple fact that honest self-analysis is seldom pleasant. In the course of any one day we all do many things which we would just as soon not remember. Consequently we shy away from them, sometimes burying them so determinedly that it takes a professional analyst to force us to face up to them. The problem then is to make your nightly self-examination honest without being morbid. You need neither berate nor excuse yourself but just honestly admit your own faults for the purpose of not repeating them. Learn to do this, and you will really be making progress. There are few areas where your new powers of concentration will help you more. For, once you learn to stay with this kind of self-examination long enough to reach realistic conclusions, you will be well on the way to true self-knowledge.

We have now seen how, beginning with simple, mechanical, physical routines, Yoga helps you to better emotional and intellectual concentration. There is yet another area where concentration can be of infinite value, and that is in matters of health. For the body, like the mind, is naturally suggestible, as any doctor with insight into psychosomatic medicine will tell you. For instance, you probably know how easy it is to develop a momentary sore throat from listening to a singer with a tight voice. Partially-deaf people often find their hearing fluctuating, depending on whether or not what is being said is something they want to hear. These reactions are so spontaneous that we have very little control over them. Conscious exercise of the mind, however, can and will counteract the unconscious impulses.

Earlier in the book we have seen how it is possible to utilize *prana*, directing it to sick areas of the body to effect cures in cases of minor ailments such as headaches and colds. This "thinking yourself well," however, cannot be accomplished without proper concentration. If the neophyte rarely succeeds in achieving beneficial results, it is because of an inherent inability to direct the *prana* currents long enough and steadfastly enough to do much good. Developing the art of single-mindness is the secret here.

When it comes to more serious illnesses such as heart disease or ulcers brought on by mental stresses and strains, arthritis and hardening of the arteries that have their basis in a person's rigidity of character, back trouble precipitated by the mental burdens one feels he is carrying—all these are syndromes which a doctor seldom conquers alone. He may help, or he may temporarily alleviate the patient's suffering. But as fast as he prescribes, the patient himself undermines the cure just so long as he persists in his initial mental attitudes. But Deep Concentration can create a new attitude just for the trying. In part it will achieve this by contributing to a more serene emotional climate. But even more importantly it will help the patient achieve insight into himself, his attitudes and blindspots. And once he understands the emotional causes of his illness he will be on the road to coping with them.

This then is how you can make a major contribution to your overall well-being, your health, your peace of mind, and finally that inner poise and purposefulness which are the foundation of better relationships with the people around you. This is how you can learn to control your immediate destinies, and so in the long run control your entire future to a great extent. Just a few minutes a day, everyday, devoted to Deep Concentration: a modest beginning indeed, but in time, with perseverance, it will truly make you the captain of your own soul, the master of your fate.

CHAPTER IX

Meditation: Final Step Toward True Self-Mastery

We have seen how Dynamic Concentration becomes the key to mastery of the mind. Consider now the purposes to which such mastery may be put—the many ways in which it can be made to work for you. In the twentieth century, with its preoccupation with the inner man, its constant questing after psychological insights, it becomes especially important and useful to each of us to be able to turn the searchlight of knowledge inward.

Using Concentration as a tool, the next, and final, step toward true self-mastery is Meditation. Yoga teaches that through Meditation the individual learns to be truly and fully conscious of himself as a unit separate and distinct from all other manifestations of life, not merely in the highly personal, individualistic Western sense, which all too often leads to egocentricity and uneasy self-absorption, but in a serene, detached way that makes him immune to superficial influences. The average person, daily subjected to competitive pressures, influenced by the fears and insecurities of others, easily becomes prey to anxiety or even panic while trying to live up to impossible standards artificially set up by his social milieu. But those few who wisely take time to find out *who they are*, quickly lose the need to play a lifelong game of "follow the leader." They learn to differentiate between what is right for them and what is not, what they really want out of life and what they have been made to *believe* they want. They learn to be true to themselves and through this awareness are liberated from conformity.

Yet as Freud and Jung and Adler have pointed out, to know one's Self, to be able to take stock without rationalization or self-delusion, is a most difficult and painful process. For in order to be completely honest in our self-appraisal we must learn to admit that we are what we are, not idealized, romanticized versions of ourselves. Often in order to achieve this we are forced to dig deep into memory for things we have allowed our conscious to forget because once they seemed humiliating or shameful to our ego. In fact, to dredge them up is so unpleasant that for most people self-examination sessions generally end up in failure. Another frequent pattern, after superficial self-analysis, is to make fine, sweeping resolutions to change and mend our ways by main force. This, as we all know, never works. Sometimes we bog down first into self-condemnation, then into self-pity. But mostly we escape by permitting our thoughts to wander away from the main problem—to let us drift a hundred dream-miles away.

How, then, are you going to be sure whether the goals you have set for yourself are your own heart's desire or the reflection of what you have been taught to consider desirable? How to tell whether your behavior patterns are truly those which suit you or have been foisted on you by circumstance? And just what is the interrelation between your external behavior and the inner problems with which you live? More specifically, what is the particular load you, as a civilized man or woman, are being forced to carry—and what can you do to lighten it?

Whether the load be emotional or physical, often the roots are the same. For instance violent headaches may be due to inadequate glasses, but may also be brought on by repressed resentments. Thus chronic migraines are frequently an expression of anger so violent that the super-ego is afraid to admit it.

The migraine sufferer presents a gentle face to the world while turning the anger inward. An ulcer case may be a man who has permitted himself to be maneuvered into a highly-paying job he hates rather than stick to the less financially rewarding but personally more gratifying work he once dreamed about. And what of the vague anxieties, the sleeplessness, the sudden fatigue most people experience at one time or another—what about that familiar inability to finish the tasks you start, or even to get started at all, because you cannot seem to overcome an ingrained conviction that you must inevitably fail, that nothing you do can possibly be good or successful?

You have doubtless recognized yourself in one or another of these descriptions. You also know perfectly well that the popular diagnosis for them all, as well as for a hundred other stumbling blocks in the path of human happiness, happens to be the correct one—it's all in the mind. Yet to bring about a change is like trying to lift yourself by your own proverbial bootstraps. The real problem eludes you. It is at this point that many people begin to consider psychoanalysis—at an average cost of $20 a fifty-minute hour.

And yet it is a fact that you yourself can change your mental attitude and remedy the physical manifestations these bring about once you learn to face and stay with your problems long enough to sort out the confusions. First you must discover what is the real 'you' in the clutter of superimposed images. Next you must decide, just as you would with an analyst's help, which of your problems you are able to do something about, and which you must learn to live with in the light of objective reality. Once you have achieved such self-knowledge you will feel you have stopped beating your head against the wall. An inner sense of serenity will replace senseless turmoil, the need to build up complicated mechanisms for camouflaging rebellion and finding escape will vanish, and you will be free to direct your energies constructively.

By now you can readily see why true Meditation—the kind taught by Yoga—requires the preparatory disciplines which can only be learned through Deep Concentration. But once you are able to stay with any one thought long enough to examine its every facet and not go on to another subject until you are ready to do so of your own volition, you have enough self-control to proceed. Actually Meditation is less stringent than concentration. In Meditation, instead of staying sternly with one point, you are free to let thoughts flow into your mind, always provided they are germane to the main subject. Of course in order to keep from drifting into aimless time-wasting day-dreaming or even free association of ideas, the Yogi does start out, as in concentration, by deliberately focusing his mind on something specific—often a part of his body. Hence the common, grossly vulgarized Western concept of Yoga Meditation as the image of a man in a turban sitting cross-legged in contemplation of his navel; nothing, it goes without saying, could be further from the truth.

To learn to control your thinking and emotions at the source, to subdue restlessness, calm the nerves and literally *will yourself* to bring out what is best in you, to shut yourself off from worry and all negative attitudes, these are the realistic goals of Meditation which you may set up for yourself. Begin with the following deceptively simple exercise: For twelve seconds, try keeping your mind on a single point—let us say the spot between the eyebrows, where the mystical "third eye" is supposed to be. Visualize that potential "third eye"; consider the benefits clairvoyance might give you, were you to achieve it; consider the uses to which seers have put their own clairvoyance. In short, meditate on every angle of the subject that suggests itself to you. Twelve seconds of such meditation is called *Dharana*. If you stay with your thought twelve times twelve seconds, permitting an unhampered flow of *related* images to come freely to mind, you have achieved *Dhyana*, or true Meditation. The Yogis teach that once you learn this you may eventually also achieve *Samadhi*, which is variously described as a state of super-consciousness and a state of infinite bliss. But *Samadhi* is not a goal for us to strive after, since it is completely alien to our own outlook.

Now for the actual procedures, the physical requirements for Meditation. To begin with, you must be alone and undisturbed when you attempt it. Therefore choose a time of day when it is easiest for you to be alone. Shut your door—lock it if necessary—to insure privacy. Be sure you are away from the phone, from loud noises, and that no one will try to speak or call to you. For if you are in the least uneasy about possible interruptions you cannot relax, and without relaxation neither Deep Concentration nor Meditation are at all possible.

You can now readily see why for most persons an early morning or late night period is the most desirable time, exactly as with most other Yoga practices. Remember you must wear completely comfortable, loose clothing, avoid the glare of bright sunshine or other light directly in your eyes and also avoid bright, disturbing décor in the room. Let the background be unobtrusive. If it should be impossible for you to settle on an appropriate spot inside your own house, try a park bench in clement weather or a library reading room in winter—any place where, in the midst of strangers, you will be left very much alone. Then the occasional sounds of the life around you will merge into the background of your consciousness. They will be much easier to shut out than the demands of your intimate, personal world.

Traditionally the Yogis prefer to meditate while sitting in one of the classic postures, or *asanas*. The *Padmasana*, or Lotus Pose, is considered ideal (see illust. Ch. XI) but the *Yoga-Mudra*, which is easier for the beginner, is equally satisfactory (Illust. page 121). Or you may sit on the floor tailor fashion. Another good position for Meditation is *Savasana*, the Death Pose—also assumed for Deep Relaxation, lying flat on your back on a hard surface, arms alongside the body. Deep Meditation in the *Savasana* pose, however, is not for those who doze off easily. It is only recommended for persons who find it too tiring or otherwise difficult to learn one of the upright positions. It goes without saying, of course, that all of these poses are only possible if you meditate in the privacy of your own room. They are obviously impossible under any other circumstances. Then too, if your time for Meditation is limited and you are unable to retire behind closed doors, you may practice it successfully while sitting comfortably in a chair; but be certain not to slump or otherwise twist your body into a position of imbalance, since this will induce restlessness and make correct breathing difficult.

Needless to say correct rhythmic breathing is essential to proper Meditation. Without it you will fail to experience that

sense of well-being and ease which frees your inner self from
the straightjacket of minor physical discomforts and distrac-
tions. As you breathe the Yoga way, you will be augmenting
the intake of *prana* so essential to both peace of mind and
health. However, rhythmic breathing should no longer be a
problem for you at this stage, nor even a matter of conscious
effort. We hope it has become a habit, but it is a good idea
to check on it.

Once you are comfortably settled in the posture you have
chosen, you may begin your meditation in one of two ways.
You may close your eyes and concentrate on the space directly
above the root of your nose—the seat of the supposedly-
atrophied Third Eye; or else, keeping your eyes open, focus
on some small article or spot directly in your line of vision.
Be sure it is something you see clearly, without straining the
eyes. Let us say you have picked a single letter in the title of a
book, printed in bold type on the dust jacket. Concentrate on
that letter until the rest of the title fades out of your consciousness. You do not have to stare so hard that your eyes begin to
sting and water—just shut everything out except the spot of
your choice. You will soon see nothing on either side, neither
words nor individual letters, only what you wish to see. You
will also, we might mention in passing, be benefiting your
eyesight; but that is what may be termed a fringe benefit.

Now that your attention has been brought under control
you are ready for the next step: Transfer your thinking gently
to the subject on which you wish to meditate. Withdraw your
thoughts from all outward contact, exactly as a tortoise draws
its head into its shell. Thus concentration will almost imper-
ceptibly merge into Meditation.

Since Meditation is very much an acquired art and takes
much practice, you will find that at first it will be easiest to
select subjects that are not too elusive. In fact, you might try
something decidedly concrete, but with a possible spiritual or
symbolic side as well. Take, for instance, the human heart.
Close your eyes and as you breathe turn your attention inward
and try to become physically aware of your pulse-beat, which

is also your heart-beat. Next visualize the heart itself: Think of it as simply a vital muscle pumping blood through the body; think of its four chambers, the valves which make the blood flow always in the same direction, of the relationship to it of the veins and arteries; of its rhythm when you are at peace and its quickened pace when excitement, physical exertion or deep emotion stimulate it; then consider the meaning of a warm heart, a generous heart, a loving heart. Gradually you will find yourself engrossed in Meditation that encompasses much broader vistas and touches upon more lofty considerations than anything which concerns one individual alone. You will feel a sense of peace taking possession of your entire being, and you will be the better for it.

Other subjects which might take you in similar manner from concrete to spiritual contemplation are: Light, beginning with a lighted candle and continuing to sunlight and enlightenment and the flow of the spirit; a book, which becomes the symbol of learning; a flower; a cloud. Later on you might choose some historical personage whom you especially admire and with whom you feel a deep sense of identity. Consider his life history, the events which led up to his greatness and what it was that made him particularly admirable; then notice how, for the moment, you are trying to view the world through the prism of his personality. This will give you an insight and an awareness of Self keener than you ordinarily experience, for in a sense it will be a shared experience. At the same time you will be able to look at yourself as if from another viewpoint. The added insight will help you disentangle your Self from identity with your mind. Such insight is one of the main objects of Meditation, since most of us have never learned to make a distinction between Self and the mind, nor do we stop to realize that they are not one and the same, Self being constant in its inherent nature, while the mind, by its very nature, is subject to endless modification.

From here on you may feel free to choose your own subjects for your daily Meditation—always making sure that you think along positive, constructive lines rather than negatively, along lines that are gloomy or self-destructive. Gradually you will discover that you are re-educating all your thought processes to work *for you*. And as the days go by and you become more adept at looking inward, you will more and more clearly learn to recognize the workings of your own mind, until you are able to dwell on whatever you wish to build up and to shut out whatever you feel needs discarding. Not only will you learn not to torture yourself with fruitless fears and worries but you will find it possible to direct your course through life, bypassing failures and choosing what is right and good for you.

Now to warn you about a few obvious pitfalls: You may start by feeling self-conscious about the entire procedure—much more so than about, say, deep breathing or concentration which are in a sense more tangible practices. If you do, try to keep in mind that this is a natural early reaction for the average Western mind. Try also to take an honest look at yourself and see whether the self-consciousness isn't a mask for laziness or for procrastination. We all have a degree of resistance against routines and disciplines, and fasten on to any excuse which presents itself. Simply refuse to accept your own excuse, however plausible it may sound. Continue practicing daily, if only for a few minutes, and soon Meditation will have become a stimulating, natural habit.

A sense of self-consciousness, of just feeling foolish about it, may also mask a lack of self-confidence. You may be convinced that you are not a "thinker" and so cannot possibly succeed. This, of course, is very far from the truth. Meditation is for anyone who stays with it; no one demands of you that you be a Spinoza or a Plato. Choose subjects that are harmonious with your own Self; make friends, so to speak, with your own mind and your own spirit.

To return once more to the rather striking parallel between Yoga Meditation and modern psychoanalysis: Analysis is largely built on the realization that knowledge of our mental mechanisms gives us insight and, more importantly, power over them; but analysts assume that in order to gain such knowledge and power we need trained help. Yoga, on the other hand, maintains that man is completely capable of doing the job himself and that he will grow, mature and become a better person in the doing if only he has the will to proceed.

It was the Greek philosopher Pythagoras who used to advise his followers to make a habit of reviewing each night their actions for that day and the day preceding it. In your quest for self-knowledge you would do well to follow the same system. But do this not in a spirit of self-flagellation, but objectively, so that having once recognized your own weaknesses you will be on the lookout for them.

Be on guard not to use your Meditation period as a whipping-post of conscience. Too often persons who are too hard on themselves during their moments of introspection unconsciously assume the attitude that, having already punished themselves, they have wiped the slate clean and are free to make the same mistakes over again. Remember that the purpose of Yoga Meditation is not punishment but serene change.

It is also *not* the purpose of Meditation to make you into a self-absorbed, egotistical person. On the contrary, your increased self-knowledge and understanding will inevitably give you increased understanding of the weaknesses and short-comings of others, so that you will be less prone to sit in judgment on your fellow-beings. Consequently your relationships with the people around you will gradually become more harmonious and warmer in quality. As your understanding of yourself deepens, as you learn not to dwell on past failures, not to give way to groundless fears or panic over trifles, you will feel free to give more of yourself to others.

Thus the self-knowledge brought about by systematic Meditation will first become the basis for greater self-reliance and self-confidence and later will help improve every human equation of which you are a part. Through Meditation you will gain a sense of perspective that will enable you to view the world around you objectively, to accept hard facts, gauge the good and the bad at their correct value and so never again allow yourself to be weighed down with a sense of impotence or defeat. Similarly there will be no room in your heart for envy, jealousy, resentment or hatred, since all these emotions stem from weakness, insecurity and fear. Instead, you will experience fresh inner strength which will be your balance wheel the rest of your life.

CHAPTER X

Why Practice Asanas?

Although a few of the specific Yoga postures, or *asanas*, have been mentioned in previous chapters, we have reversed the usual procedure followed in handbooks on Yoga, postponing their general discussion until now in order to let the student first acquire a good overall grasp of the subject. For the *asanas* are meaningful only in conjunction with the other Yoga practices with which they are both physically and spiritually interrelated. An unthinking approach could easily reduce them to a set of tricks for the double-jointed, and their apparent difficulty discourage the neophyte before he ever gives himself a chance to see what he can do and especially what the *asanas* can do *for him*.

In the next chapter we shall go into specific descriptions of those postures which the Western student may safely attempt without a teacher. We shall describe them in minute detail and explain step by step how to do them accurately; and also list the physical benefits derived from each one. In that way each student will be able not only to appreciate their meaning and importance, but also be in a better position to decide for himself which ones are suited to his needs and should be incorporated into his daily routine, and which may be either omitted or done only occasionally as time permits and inclination warrants.

Indian legend claims that the god Shiva originally demonstrated 84,000 postures and exercises for maintaining health and attaining self-discipline. Patanjali, the father of Yoga, when codifying its theory in his famous Yoga Sutras, reduced the essential number of *asanas* to 84—the number in common use in India today. But this number is for Yoga disciples who devote their full lives to this pursuit. Only about twenty to thirty *asanas* may be considered easily adaptable to Occidental usage, and, even then, one must bear in mind that "easily" here is a relative term and that it will require considerable patience and perseverance to achieve most of the ones we shall describe. This, however, need not discourage you. In the first place, regular practice will do wonders in developing your body and stretching and limbering up lazy muscles. In the second place, you must never overtax yourself; if an exercise really seems too difficult or seems to result in serious strain, abandon it immediately. You may then either return to it at a later date or, guiding yourself by your own instinct for what seems best for you, abandon it altogether. Always remember you are not in competition either with yourself or with anyone else. Do only what seems feasible to you. Regularity and a proper approach are more important than feats of prowess. In fact the latter aren't considered in the least desirable as part of Yoga.

When Patanjali was writing his Sutras he was not only writing for contemporaries but for experts—persons already deeply versed in the science and philosophy of Yoga and the art of Meditation and body culture. Hence the traditional descriptions of the *asanas*, as well as statements regarding their therapeutic values, are masterpieces of condensation and economy. For centuries they have been passed down from *Guru* to *chela* in something like shorthand, comprehensible only to the initiate. The Western reader approaching the subject cold might see only a jumble of fantastic claims like those of a witch doctor. For this reason we are including here a brief discussion of the physiology of the *asanas* as related to physiology in general. Viewed from this angle the entire subject becomes quickly comprehensible in common-sense terms. And here it is interesting to note that as recently as the turn of the century Occidental medical science shrugged off *asanas* as so much mysticism. Today this attitude has altered considerably. The reason is that Western medicine has finally succeeded in explaining in language satisfactory to itself the benefits which the human body derives from Hindu practices. Having thus established their *raison d'etre*, their scientific rationale, it no longer feels in honor bound to scoff.

Some of the postures we shall describe are referred to as *mudras :* these are the purely static poses recommended purely for meditation and relaxation and also sometimes for breathing or *pranayama*. The *asanas*—sometimes also referred to as exercises because in order to attain them a certain amount of effort and motion are necessary—are those postures which directly benefit the physical organism. One of the salient differences between *asanas* and our own idea of physical exercise is that in all Yogi exercise there is a minimum of motion involved, with everything done at a slow tempo. This, of course, is the direct opposite of Western calisthenics, gymnastics and sports in general, all of which require speed and drilling.

In order to be healthy the body needs to keep its cells and tissues in perfect condition. This in turn requires regular feeding, which is not the same as having regular meals. Many of us who eat quite regularly simply do not get enough benefit out of the food we swallow and enjoy. For unless food is properly digested and assimilated with the aid of well-functioning endocrine gland secretions and oxygen it does little good and sometimes even harms us, as when it turns to surplus fat instead of to energy. Similarly, after it has been digested there is waste, which must be rapidly and thoroughly eliminated via the bowels, kidneys and sweat glands. Here again improper functioning of the organs or a malfunctioning of the endocrines may cause trouble. Lastly, in order to feel well we must have healthy, alert nerves serving both the central and the sympathetic nervous system. The human body that functions properly in all three of these departments will then result in a clear head and an alert, well-functioning brain.

Only a healthy digestive and circulatory system can do the work of breaking down the foods we eat and so supply the tissues with the proteins, fats, minerals, sugar and carbohydrates we require. But civilized man's physical deterioration begins early in life and the processes necessary to keep the body in condition tend to slow up all too soon. Moreover, since we were once quadrupeds, the architecture of the human body is quite ill-adapted to our upright position. We simply aren't built to last and wear well. So it is that with the years our back stiffens or develops curvatures; internal organs drop; women's breasts sag and men have a tendency to hernia. All this is the result of our walking upright. In addition we face such problems as middle-age fat due to uneven metabolic action, calcium deposits in the joints producing arthritis and a number of other by-products of the aging process—conditions already mentioned earlier.

As you know, the digestive organs—the stomach, small intestine, pancreas and liver—depend for health in part at least on the proper functioning of the abdominal muscles, specifically of the diaphragm. For as the diaphragm rises and falls with breathing, the organs in the upper abdominal cavity receive regular massage at the rate of some forty to fifty strokes a minute. But the average city dweller's breathing is so shallow, his abdominal muscles so flabby, that the massage does not really accomplish what it is supposed to. Stomach acid is then secreted improperly and digestion suffers. This in turn may result in minor disturbances such as gas or "acid stomach," or it may lead to more serious disorders. But with the regular practice of appropriate *asanas* the abdominal muscles readily regain their elasticity and tone. Other *asanas* will have a similarly beneficial effect on the muscles of the back and on the internal back muscles within the abdominal cavity. Between them, these will restore the over-civilized stomach to proper functioning. Naturally *asanas* begun while the body is perfectly healthy will be insurance against future trouble.

In addition to promoting proper digestion, *asanas* designed to strengthen the abdominal walls also keep the internal organs within the abdomen in their proper place. In this way prolapse of the stomach, intestines, kidneys, uterus or male reproductive organs may easily be avoided. An added benefit which we certainly must not minimize is that strong abdominal muscles add to the beauty and grace of the human body: and who wouldn't rather achieve a good figure by this pleasant means than with the help of tight girdles and surgical belts!

Proper circulation, indispensable for carrying food particles from digestive organs to tissues, is also a matter of strong muscles, since the heart itself is basically a giant muscle constantly at work. All the *asanas* which have an effect on the diaphragm help massage the heart at the same time as they massage the abdominal organs. They achieve this by subjecting the heart to alternate pressures. On the other hand, the reverse postures—like the Headstand and the Plough—also have a special beneficial effect on the veins, since during those *asanas* the blood is made to flow back to the heart without effort, considerably reducing normal pressures and giving the veins a rest they would not normally get even when the body is prone. Yogis claim that with perseverance even varicose veins may be cured by this method. Certainly they can be helped and even more certainly prevented.

Pranayama practiced alone is in itself extremely beneficial to the lungs and hence to the proper cleansing of the blood. But *pranayama* practiced in conjunction with certain *asanas* will even further strengthen thoracic muscles and, again through subjecting them to alternating pressures, increase the elasticity of the lung tissues. At the same time it will have a cleansing effect on the air passages, leaving you less susceptible to colds and tonsilitis. In fact, whenever a cold threatens or you detect signs of incipient tonsilitis, practicing *pranayama* and the proper *asanas*, especially the Lion Pose, will have an immediate therapeutic effect: the illness will be nipped in the bud.

Ordinary exercise seldom has any direct bearing on the proper functioning of the endocrine glands but—again through the subtle effect of certain positions and motions—many of the *asanas* will stimulate the functioning of one or another set of endocrines. Similarly, there are *asanas* for stimulating the proper functioning of the kidneys, the large intestine and the colon. Often the specific desired effect is obtained by some slight pressure, some stretch or twist of the body or a position which sets otherwise seldom-used tendons and sinews into play. Since for reasons of space it is obviously impossible here to analyze the anatomical aspects of each *asana* in detail, you yourself might, if your mind has this kind of inquisitive turn, try figuring out the physiological reasons for each claim. If you study the anatomical charts as well as the *Chakras* on pages 58–59, you can readily work out the relationship of the postures to the various organs and glands in the body. In each case you will then discover that the relationship, and therefore the effect on the general well-being of the body, is a very direct one. Once you have gained such understanding you will come closer to the Yogi's own ability to fill in the shorthand indications of what each pose will do. The claims in terms of added health and strength will become clear to you, and they will no longer seem extravagant.

As we consider the benefits of various *asanas* on the nervous system—certainly it becomes obvious how improved circulation and digestion directly affect the health of the nerves—we begin also to understand that this effect is more than a purely physical one. A better supply of blood to the brain inevitably results in improved memory, alertness, an overall improvement in one's mental attitudes and a revitalization of all the faculties. A person's whole outlook is therefore affected by what in the beginning is a series of physical exercises. So there is nothing mystical or mysterious in the claim that Yoga *asanas* have a direct bearing on the human mind and spirit.

In practicing them it is important to remember that, if we want them to be completely effective, the *asanas* must always be approached in a peaceful state of mind. Otherwise the healing forces they liberate are squandered in neutralizing disturbed emotions rather than being used to calm the nerves and produce a heightened state of well-being. The best way to begin one's daily practice, then, is with a few Dynamic Breathing exercises followed by a meditative pose, or *mudra*, which will help induce the proper calm state of mind. You should always strive to set aside the problems that beset you, filling your mind instead with thoughts of peace and serenity, turning your eyes inward and away from the materialistic world.

Finally, a word of caution: In choosing the exercises which you feel are right for you, you should be guided by the knowledge that anyone who takes the time and trouble to observe the reactions of his own organism will soon be able to tell as instinctively as a healthy animal which of them are likely to be beneficial and which might prove harmful. So be selective as you set up your routine and never be afraid to trust your own judgment. There is no need to follow the book slavishly; in fact, if *asanas* exhaust you because of health or age reasons you may find it best merely to do Deep Relaxation and Breathing routines, or perhaps confine your *asanas* at first to *Savasana*, recommended for Deep Relaxation. No matter how little the exertion, you will begin to benefit if you practice regularly, day after day, in the proper frame of mind. In time it is quite possible that the relaxation itself, as well as correct breathing, will envigorate your body to the point where you are ready to try something more complicated. But under no circumstances must you continue Yoga exercises beyond the point of tiredness.

Our final caution is to emphasize how important it is to follow whatever specific warnings may be included in the descriptions. For instance, if it is mentioned that a certain *asana* is not recommended for persons in a category to which you belong, just forget about it. There are surely others which you can substitute. Always remember to rest and do a few breathing exercises between *asanas*. Above all, remember that your own frame of mind is what will determine the final success of your endeavor.

CHAPTER XI

Basic Asanas
(Postures and Exercises)

Of the 22 *asanas* described in this chapter, you may only be able to execute two, three or four. This is not of too great importance. As we have said again and again, Yoga is not a system of mere body culture, and since you are not in competition with yourself, you need not be disturbed or discouraged at any point simply because you cannot do at once what you are trying to do while practicing. Of course, with patience you may be able to improve steadily and limber up as time goes on, and be the better for it, but this after all is not your main purpose. Always keep in mind that what really counts in the daily routine you establish for yourself is the fusing of mental, spiritual and physical experience. You want to learn to live at full capacity, and not to drive yourself beyond that capacity.

That is not to say that if the description of a certain *asana* sounds exactly like what the doctor ordered, but seems at first all but unfeasible, you should not try to incorporate it into your schedule even though it requires effort. Work at it by all means, but approach your task with plenty of patience and perseverance. It does not matter if at first you cannot do it properly, for like any other routine it will become easier and easier with repetition. Stiff muscles and joints will gradually limber up. Only be sure not to dissipate your energies: it is better to practice a single *asana* morning and night for a while, perfecting it before you go on to another one, than to go through a dozen exercises sloppily and without due thought.

Almost all Westerners, except athletes and the very young or very limber, find their joints protesting painfully when they begin Yoga practice. In addition, sitting for even a few minutes in a fixed position will make your limbs ache. This is only natural, and when this happens, simply stretch briefly, gently massage the aching spot, then resume the position. At the end of a week you will find the whole procedure a good deal easier.

At the risk of being repetitive, let us remind you again that all *asanas* should be done in conjunction with deep rhythmic breathing and with complete concentration. Remember to rest briefly after each *asana*. It is always best to plan to alternate the more envigorating ones with the completely restful; for instance, after the Headstand, the Savasana; after the Plough, the Lotus Pose, and so on. Since the control of consciousness is your ultimate goal, it goes without saying that it is all-important to concentrate deeply on what you are doing. Only in this manner will your mind be exerting maximum influence on every single muscle and tendon, every nerve and blood cell, while at the same time your rhythmic breathing will be filling your body with *prana*—charging it, so to speak, with the positive vital currents so essential to health, healing and long life.

Always begin your exercises with a period of Deep Relaxation followed by the breathing routines given in Chapter V. Set aside a fixed time for them each day. Morning is probably best, in which case the exercises should be done immediately upon getting up, before breakfast but after your cleansing routines. Preferably the bowels should be moved beforehand, but this may not be feasible for you, since so many people habitually do not have a bowel movement until after breakfast. Do not become unduly concerned with this last point—simply make it a practice to use the toilet at a regular time; and eventually your habits will change.

If you choose to do your Yoga exercises before retiring at night, make certain you are not over-tired, but fully enough awake to relax and concentrate on what you are doing. Obviously little benefit would be derived from either *asanas* or *mudras* performed while the mind is in such a state of fatigue that it cannot address itself to the task at hand. Without the proper mental mood the routines become so many physical exercises, an exotic but ineffectual substitute for calisthenics.

Remember that all Yoga exercises should be performed on the hard floor, using a rug or mat for protection. A mattress or soft bed is inadvisable since you would not derive the maximum muscular benefits from exercising on a "giving" surface.

The *asanas* listed are not given in any order that must be strictly followed, although to some extent they progress from relatively simple ones to those more complicated. Nor will you be expected to do them all. Few Westerners have the time to devote to such concentrated training. It will be up to you to choose those exercises which suit your individual needs and purposes, or which appeal to you. However, just as the Yogis generally begin with a period of meditation, so you too might find it advisable to start with a simple pose. Finally, bear in mind that you are always free to alter any already-established routine, adding or cutting down as you see fit.

1. SAVASANA, or the *Death Pose*, already described in Chapter VI; this is the pose of complete relaxation.

Method : Let yourself lie flat and heavy on the mat. Breathe rhythmically but naturally. Try to *feel* the weight of your body as though it were digging into the ground. Consciously relax every muscle, starting with the head, neck, shoulders, chest, arms and hands and fingers, down the torso and abdomen, down the back, hips, thighs, knees, legs, feet and toes. Relax the muscles of your face—forehead, eyes, cheeks, mouth, chin. Pretend you are an old piece of rope lying on the ground. When you have relaxed com-

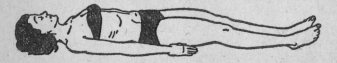

pletely, repeat the process. You will discover a residue of tension here and there which must be gotten rid of. Do not let your mind wander and free-associate, but concentrate on some soothing image, such as clouds floating in the sky. Hold the image. Do not let yourself relax into sleep. After a few moments reverse the process by deliberately tensing the relaxed muscles one by one. Stretch hard. In time you should be able to hold this pose for ten or fifteen minutes without either day-dreaming or falling asleep. You will find such relaxation more beneficial than an hour's nap.

2. UDHITTA PADASANA, or *Raised-Legs Posture*, is a simple *asana* which may be done by anyone, regardless of age, weight or infirmities, and is therefore excellent for the beginner.

Method : Lie flat on your back, arms along the sides as for SAVASANA. Inhaling slowly, slowly raise your right leg without bending the knee, until it is at right angles to your body, keeping your other leg flat on the floor. Hold this position for a few seconds, then lower the leg while exhaling in the same slow rhythm. Reverse, repeating with the left leg. Now raise both legs at once. Hold this position for a slow count of three times three (counting to three in waltz time approximates one second) and lower the legs again. Rest. Gradually increase the count to ten or twelve seconds.

At first you may find that doing the three parts of this exercise just once is enough to produce slight fatigue. But after a few days you will be able to increase the number of repetitions to three, then four or five. Eventually you should be able to raise

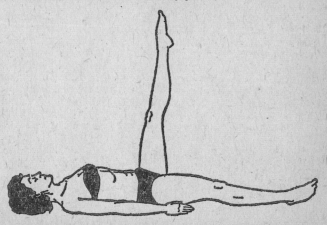

both legs at once half a dozen times in smooth rhythm without stopping. Be sure, however, always to go through all motions *slowly :* the tendency is to lower the legs fast, since this is by far the easier way. You will probably experience slight soreness of the abdominal muscles at the start, but this will not last beyond the first few days.

Therapeutic Value : This exercise gives the abdomen an internal massage, strengthening all the muscles and breaking down surplus fat. It is therefore particularly good for persons working at sedentary jobs and for those suffering from or wishing to prevent "middle-aged spread," including women who otherwise depend on girdles to keep themselves looking flat. It is excellent for preventing prolapse of the stomach and for reconditioning muscles after childbirth. In the latter case, however, it should not be done without first checking with a doctor.

Caution : This exercise should be avoided by persons with a weak heart and women already suffering from female disorders.

In contrast with the above *asanas*, which are basically Deep Contraction exercises, the next three are Concentration Poses. They are listed in the logical order in which you will want to do them, the first being the simplest and the last the most complicated. But even the first will require a bit of patience at first, unless you are naturally very limber.

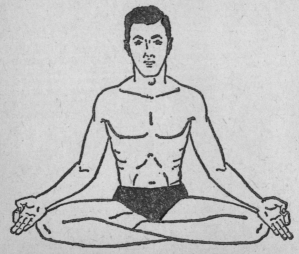

3. SUKHASANA, also called the *Simple Pose :*
Method : Sit on the mat with legs stretched out in front. Bend

the right leg at the knee and place the foot under the left thigh, using your hands to do it. Now bend the left leg and place the left foot under the right leg. (You may, if you wish, reverse the order in which the legs are bent. Left-handed persons will generally find themselves naturally doing this in regard to many positions). Keep the body balanced and easily erect. Extend your arms so that the wrists rest on your knees, palms turned upward. The tips of the thumbs should touch the tips of the index fingers, with other fingers lying straight out.

At first your knees will persist in sticking up into the air, which is only natural, since unlike the Orientals we have no tradition of sitting cross-legged unless our ancestors were tailors! You may find it helpful to start practicing this seated on a large book about two inches thick. Do not force the knees down. Eventually you will be able to achieve this pose with ease and will assume it naturally for meditation.

Therapeutic Value : This exercise helps concentration and induces mental and physical stability through calming the nervous system.

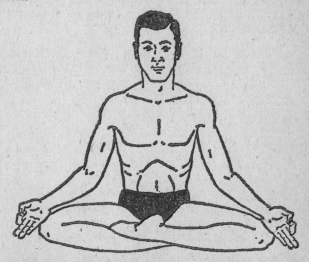

4. SIDDHASANA, the *Advanced* or *Perfect Pose :*

Method : Having mastered the Simple Pose, you are now ready to go on to the Advanced Pose, and you will find that your abilities of concentration become much greater. Superficially there is considerable similarity between the two exercises, and you begin the SIDDHASANA as you do the SUKHASANA. This time, however, you start sitting upright, tailor fashion, then take the left foot in the right hand and bend it so that the left heel is placed against the perineum (the structure between the genitals and the anus) and the sole of the left foot touches the upper portion of the right thigh. Be careful not to sit *on* the heel, which should just feel the two bones of the perineum. Now bend the right leg so that the right heel is against the pubic bone and the toes of the right foot fit snugly into the crevice formed by the calf and thigh of the left leg. Next, place your left hand, palm upward, on your left knee and the right hand on the right knee. Keep the head erect, pressing your chin well into your neck. Close your eyes and begin to concentrate by focusing your imagination on a spot between your eyebrows. This is not a must; but your mind is likely to wander at first unless you do.

Therapeutic Value : Same as SUKHASANA, with increased powers of concentration.

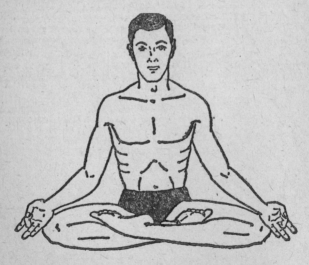

5. PADMASANA, the *Lotus* or *Buddha Pose*, one of the basic Asana and the one most Westerners will recognize as the classic Yoga pose. Of the three meditation poses it is the most difficult to achieve. But since it is also the most beneficial, by all means try eventually to train your body to assume it.

Method : Sit on the mat tailor fashion. With your hands, bring the right foot up to rest on the left thigh, close to the hip joint, with the sole of the foot upturned and the heel near the middle of the abdomen, the ball of the foot almost in line with the thigh. Now take the left foot, cross it over the right and place it in a similar position on the right thigh. (For left-handed persons, reverse the order). Place the hands on the knees, palms open, the thumb and second finger of each hand forming the letter O.

Because the Lotus Pose sometimes takes months of practice for the Occidental to achieve, many teachers advocate the following preliminary exercise:

Place the sole of your left foot against the right thigh, then begin a bouncing up-and-down movement with your left knee. You will find that the moment you push the knee down to the floor it will bounce up again like rubber—this is true even of the Simple Pose—and the bouncing routine helps stretch and limber unused tendons and ligaments. Bounce first one knee, then the other.

Therapeutic Value : The Lotus Pose, which symbolizes mental purity and a completely developed consciousness, is said to free the mind of temptations and lower physical instincts. Its perfect symmetry gives the body inner harmony, preserves the equilibrium of our positive and negative currents and increases the effect of our breathing exercises. Creative energy is said to waken like a great river dammed up so that its rising waters may be harnessed. Its immediate physical benefits are to keep the joints flexible and to promote good posture.

Perhaps you are wondering why such difficult postures as the last three are recommended for concentration, since it would seem that in order simply to concentrate one might just as well lie down and relax. Actually, this is not the case. Experience has shown that if one lies down to concentrate or meditate, it is all too easy to day-dream, drowse or even fall asleep. Standing positions, on the other hand, make it impossible to relax sufficiently for the mind to be completely free to devote itself to meditation. Over the centuries Yogis have found that the sitting posture is infinitely the superior one, and so have adopted it.

6. VIPARITAKARANI MUDRA, or the *Reverse Posture,* important because it is said to reverse not only the position of the body but also of time. Because of the way we receive radiations from both

earth and cosmic spaces, the Yogis claim that while standing on our feet we grow old, in assuming the inverted pose we grow younger.

Method : Lie flat on the back. Inhaling slowly, raise your legs upward; then, supporting your hips with your hands, gradually raise the trunk until it rests on the shoulder-blades. The knees should be straight, the legs and toes inclined slightly beyond the head. Breathe in and out deeply and slowly several times, then return to the prone position. Continue breathing deeply until all trace of effort has disappeared.

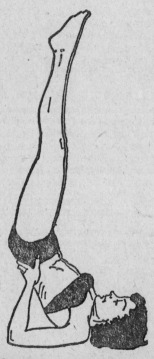

Therapeutic Value : This exercise, which really requires very little effort, is particularly beneficial because it reverses and increases the flow of blood to the head and respiratory organs. Hence it is excellent for helping cure colds and tonsilitis. It is also known as a great boon to those who wish to restore their youth and vitality, for it helps keep the endocrine glands and internal organs, as well as the skin, in youthful shape. Indian women practice it to prevent early wrinkles and general aging, and also to prevent and cure irregular or painful menstruation and the mental and physical discomforts of menopause. Men, too, find it beneficial, since it is one of the important ways to keep the gonads functioning properly.

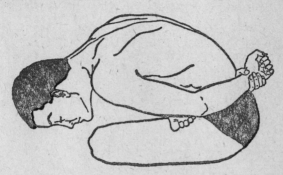

7. YOGA MUDRA, or *Symbol of Yoga*, is another posture which, while not an exercise, is considered of great spiritual value. On the other hand it also has definite physical benefits, since it promotes good elimination and so helps the system stay clean. It may be practiced between any two more strenuous poses.

Method : Sit as for the Lotus Pose, or simply tailor fashion. Now clench your fists and place them on either side of the abdomen, slightly below the navel. Take a deep breath, then bend forward as far as possible while exhaling. Continue firmly to press the fists against the abdomen. Hold this pose for five to ten seconds, retaining your breath. Now start slowly exhaling, sit up and turn to the original posture. Gradually increase the time until the Mudra takes three minutes, being careful not to add more than a second or two per week to your time. Otherwise holding the breath too long may be harmful. (The classical manner of doing this Mudra is in the Lotus Pose, with the hands behind the back, left fist clenched and right hand grasping the left wrist).

Therapeutic Value : The YOGA MUDRA increases the peristaltic movements of the bowels and so is excellent for relief of constipation. It also strengthens the abdominal muscles and lends tone to the colon, the pelvic region and the nervous system in general. Men troubled with seminal weakness are helped by it, and in advanced stages of Yoga practice it helps awaken the Kundalini power. These benefits are additional to the major one of increased concentration.

8. SIMHASANA, or the *Lion Pose*, particularly useful for relaxing the throat.

Method : Squat on your heels, or even sit in a chair for this one; place your hands on your knees, take a deep breath, exhale and stick your tongue out as far as possible, until you begin to experience a slight gagging sensation. Stiffen the fingers and spread

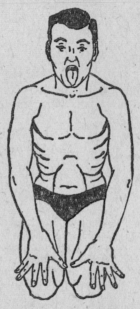

them wide. At the same time open both mouth and eyes wide, tensing the neck and throat. Let the feeling of tension permeate your whole body. Retain this posture for a few seconds, then relax. Repeat two or three times. If you feel you are coming down with a sore throat or laryngitis, repeat the exercise half a dozen times several times a day.

Therapeutic Value : The Lion Pose helps the throat by increasing the blood supply to it, so that it is better able to resist infection. At the same time the muscles and ligaments of the area are toned and the entire body benefits. This is an excellent exercise for persons suffering from asthma, hay fever, enlarged or infected tonsils, and from general susceptibility to throat and upper-respiratory infections. It is, of course, invaluable to singers and public speakers.

9. USTRASANA or *Camel Pose*, the backward-bending exercise:

Method : Kneel on the mat, then squat on the heels with toes outstretched; place the hands behind you directly behind the toes. Lean back, throwing the head as far back as possible. On a deep inhalation, slowly raise the buttocks and the lower part of the body, arching the spine. Hold the breath while retaining this position for a few seconds, then return to the original sitting position. Move the head forward and exhale. Rest and repeat, gradually

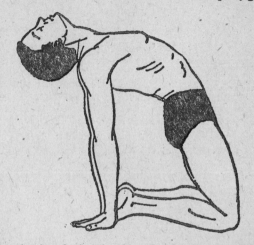

increasing the time for holding from six to thirty seconds. In time you will want to repeat this exercise up to five times a day.

Therapeutic Value : The Camel Pose benefits the thyroid and the gonads or sex glands. At the same time it lends elasticity to the spine and back muscles. Excellent for persons suffering from gas, constipation, slight displacement of the vertebrae or of the various pelvic organs such as the uterus, Fallopian tubes, ureter and urethra, and for disorders of the urinary bladder. By toning the entire pelvic area and stimulating the sex glands the Camel Pose is especially beneficial in increasing sexual potency.

Caution : Not to be attempted by persons suffering from hernia.

10. MATSYASANA, or *Fish Pose :*

Method : Starting with the Lotus Pose, lean back, using elbows and arms to help balance yourself, until your head rests comfortably on the mat and your body forms a lower arc. Use a low cushion for comfort at first, if necessary. Now extend your arms and grasp your toes on either side.

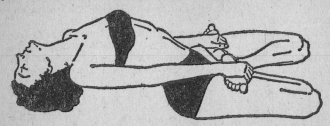

Therapeutic Value : This exercise tones every muscle in the system, especially those of the lubro-sacral region. The consciousness in the meantime is directed toward the thyroid. This pose helps overcome stiffness and tension in the neck, revitalizing neck muscles by setting up tensions opposite to the usual ones. The backward pressure stimulates the blood flow to the neck, cleansing the thyroid, tonsils and adenoids. Excellent for colds and upper-respiratory troubles, especially those of the pharynx.

11. THE SUPINE POSE, which is a variation on the Fish Pose, is considerably easier for the neophyte since it is done without crossing the legs. You might try it during the early stages of your Yoga Practice.

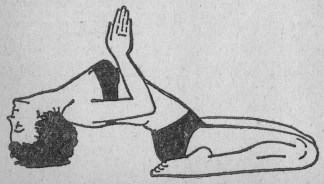

Method : Kneel on the mat, keeping knees together and feet apart, with heels up. Sitting *between* your heels, bend backward exactly as for the Fish Pose until your head rests on the floor. Fold the palms of your hands in the middle of your chest as for prayer. Hold this position for a few seconds, breathing deeply. Now raise yourself slowly, using first the elbows and arms, then the palms. Relax. Gradually increase the time of the exercise to thirty seconds.

Therapeutic Value : Both the Fish Pose and the Supine Pose benefit the pituitary, pineal, thyroid and adrenal glands as well as the gonads. They also tone the kidneys, stomach and intestines. Excellent for toning the nerves connected with sexual functions.

12. SARVANGASANA, or the *Shoulder Stand*. The name of this *asana* is derived from the Sanskrit word *sarvanga*, meaning "all parts" and implies that it is beneficial for the entire body. In performing it you will find your entire muscular structure being stretched, healed and revitalized while at the same time your powers of concentration improve. In many ways the Sarvangasana is similar to the Reverse Posture, as you will see.

Method : Lie flat on your back, legs outstretched, arms parallel to the body, palms down. Now raise the legs slowly from the floor, keeping the knees straight and close together, toes pointing. Continue the movement as slowly as possible until the legs are at a thirty-degree angle with the floor. This is Stage One. Pause briefly, breathing naturally and concentrating your whole attention on the movement.

During Stage Two, continue the elevation until your legs are vertical to your body. Pause again, maintaining the full stretch.

For Stage Three, press your hands and elbows hard on the floor and raise your legs, torso, hips, back, stomach and chest. Then, using only your upper arms and elbows as a floor rest, slide your hands up the small of the back to assist in balancing the trunk. Your legs will swing past the vertical point at this stage.

Now, for Stage Four, tuck your chin into your neck and give your body an extra lift to stretch the trunk and legs to a vertical position. Retain this pose for a few moments : you are now holding the Pan-physical Pose or Candle Posture, another classic of Hatha Yoga. Now reverse the order of your movements and *slowly* return to the original horizontal position. Rest.

Remember that at all stages your movements should be slow, smooth and controlled and that a full stretch of the entire body must be maintained throughout. In time you will be able to retain the Stage Four position for several minutes without experiencing the slightest discomfort. Always begin the descent before you are too tired to perform it on one smooth, controlled motion.

Actually this *asana* is simpler to do than to describe. But if you are one of those persons who become dizzy the moment you are turned upside down, you may need to get used to it gradually.

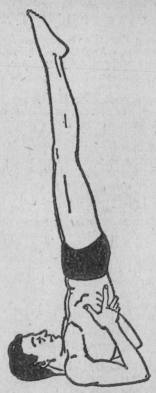

If such is the case, practice one stage at a time until you have become used to it; then go to the next. Never rush for results. Your best gauge is your own common sense.

Therapeutic Value : This *asana*, like the Reverse Pose and the Headstand (to be described later) is believed to revitalize the thyroid, which in turn affects the healthy functioning of the whole organism. It reverses the flow of blood and sends it away from the limbs and abdomen toward the head, thus relieving fatigue and easing venous congestion—hence its efficacy in leg and stomach troubles. The added flow of blood to the neck and upper body stimulate the endocrine secretions in general. At the same time the muscles of the legs, thighs, hips, abdomen, shoulders, spine, neck and arms are all stretched, adding to the suppleness of the body as a whole and improving appearance. Most importantly, the spine and the nervous system benefit so that inner tensions and irritation subside. It follows that the Shoulder Stand is of the greatest value to persons engaged in mental or creative effort.

Other benefits include relief from constipation, intestinal and digestive disorders, menstrual discomfort, hemorrhoids and varicose veins.

Caution : This *asana* should be practiced sparingly by persons suffering from chronic catarrh and should never be attempted by those with disorders of the thyroid.

13. PADHASTRASANA, or Contraction in a Standing Position:
Method : Stand erect with the legs close together. Inhale and exhale rhythmically a number of times. Finally exhale fully, and

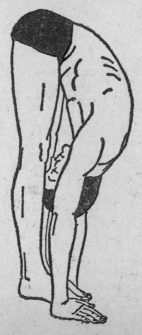

while doing this and keeping the knees stiff, bend the body until your hands reach down to your toes and your nose touches your knees. This will be difficult at first, but with patience you will find yourself able literally to bury your face between your knees and place the palms of your hands flat on the floor. Retain this bent position for five seconds, then return to the erect posture, inhaling as you straighten out. Relax. Slowly increase the time for holding to thirty seconds. Do only once.

Therapeutic Value : This is a fine slimming exercise, excellent for the waistline. It relieves constipation and loosens the muscles. Superficially it has been adapted to Western exercise, but its true value lies not in automatic repetition: it should be done only once, very slowly and dynamically, with the maximum stretch possible. It strengthens the abdominal organs, relieving dyspepsia. Its toning effect on the legs and back is excellent insurance against sciatica.

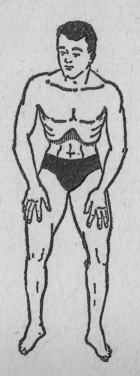

14. UDDIYANA-BANDA, or *Stomach Lift :*

Method : Stand with the knees slightly bent and place your hands, palm down, on your thighs. Breathe in and out, regularly and rhythmically, but more forcibly and longer each time. Finally exhale and continue to do so until every particle of air has been expelled from the lungs. Now raise the chest high and push out. A vacuum has been created inside your lungs and stomach. As you raise your chest, the atmospheric pressure will push your stomach flat until it all but pushes against your spine. Retain this pose for five seconds, then inhale. Repeat once only.

Therapeutic Value : This is one of the most effective exercises known for treating constipation and other digestive complaints. It is not difficult unless you happen to have a specially flabby stomach or suffer from obesity. If so, you will be doubly benefited in time, for as you continue with the Stomach Lift your muscles will be greatly strengthened and the fat will begin to melt. This

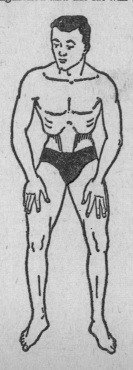

exercise should always be done in the morning on an empty stomach. It must never be attempted less than two hours after a meal.

After you have been doing the Uddiyana-Banda for several days, try drawing up your intestine while raising your chest after exhalation. This will require considerable effort. Retain this position for five seconds, relax and repeat once more. When you are able to accomplish this without effort, increase retention time to ten, twenty and even sixty seconds. However, be sure to inhale and relax the moment you feel the slightest strain. Better still, relax just as you begin to think you will feel fatigue if you continue. In time you will be able to do this exercise while sitting in the Lotus Pose.

15. NAULI-KRIYA, an advanced abdominal exercise recommended mainly for men students, to be attempted after the stomach has been made fit and supple by performance of Uddiyana-Banda and other simpler *asanas*, and after surplus fat or distention have been overcome.

Method : Stand or sit in the same position as for Uddiyana-Banda and exhale forcibly through the mouth after a few preliminary rhythmic breathing routines. Be sure all the air has been expelled from the lungs on a forcible exhalation. Raise the chest and draw the intestine up and in. Now, contract the abdominal muscles—the two recti—and arch them forward with a push. Try to isolate first the right, then the left rectus, making them stand out pillar-like, then rotating them first clockwise, then counterclockwise. This rolling action will be facilitated if you bend the trunk slightly toward one side, then the other. Roll the two recti alternately for several rotations.

Try this exercise standing at first, and once you feel confident in its performance try it in the Lotus Pose. But be sure to approach it gradually. Men over fifty, very young boys and women should not attempt it unless accustomed to hard physical exercise.

Therapeutic Value : The above two exercises are considered by experts to be the best method for keeping the abdomen fit and the intestines in perfect condition. Those who practice Uddiyana-Banda and Nauli-Kriya regularly never suffer from digestive or other intestinal disorders. The Nauli is also said to prevent nocturnal emission of semen.

16. ARDJA-MATSYENDRASANA, named after the Yogi teacher Matsyendra, is the only exercise of its kind, since it strengthens the backbone through a twisting movement on either side. It is a variation on the original movement, too difficult for the Western

student to contemplate; even so it may prove difficult for the beginner and will require patient application.

Method : Sit on the mat or rug with legs outstretched, holding the trunk erect. Then, cross your right foot over your left knee and place it flat on the floor, next to your left knee. Place the fingers of your left hand on top of the toes of your right foot.

This is the first stage of this Deep Contraction exercise. For Stage Two, stretch the left arm and grip the toes of the right foot. Place your right arm across your back so that the hand, with palm outward, rests on the waistline near the left hip. As you do this, your torso will be turned half-right. Hold this position, stretching consciously, for a few seconds. Check to see that the chest is erect, otherwise you will not get the full benefit of the *asana*. Relax. Repeat, reversing the motions, bending the right leg, and so on, and finally turning half-left. Relax again. Increase the stretch by one second every time you do this exercise, until you are able to hold the position for a full minute. Always remember that your motions must be smooth, gradual, and never jerky.

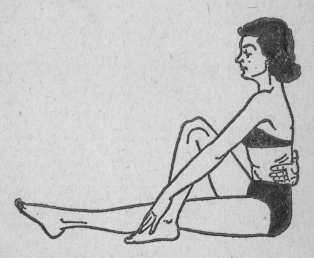

Therapeutic Value : This *asana* helps keep the spine supple and in perfect health, in addition to massaging the abdominal organs. Consequently it will relieve, and even more importantly prevent, lumbago and muscular rheumatism, as well as guard against slipped disks. Since it places pressure upon the spleen, liver and kidneys, it eliminates their sluggishness. It also helps tone the entire nervous system, acting to rejuvenate the whole body. Consequently it is considered one of the most useful of *asanas*.

17. VAKRASANA, or *Twisting Posture*, a simpler variation of the previous exercise, is done as follows:

Method : Sit on the floor with both legs stretched out straight, draw right leg up until the thigh and knee press hard against the abdomen and chest. Lift the right foot over the left and place its sole flat on the floor against the left thigh. Twist the torso to the right and place the palm of the right hand on the floor, with fingers outward, so that the body is balanced. Hold this position the length of three Yogi breaths. Relax. Reverse, then relax once more. This position may be varied by bending the outstretched leg under, and by turning the torso more definitely sideways.

Therapeutic Value : The Vakrasana has the same value as the Ardja-Matsyendrasana, but is milder. Part of its benefit is said to be derived from bringing the positive and negative currents in

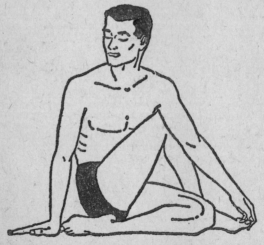

the body into equilibrium. It helps build self-confidence, determination and perseverance—literally "strengthening the backbone" in a figurative as well as a physical manner.

18. DHANURASANA, or *Bow Posture*, celebrated for its rejuvenating effects and the relaxing of many little-used muscles.

Method : Lie flat on the mat, face down, arms by your sides, both stretched taut, then bend the legs at the knees as far back as possible and catch the ankles with the corresponding hands. Pull the feet well down. Now lift the knees and thighs off the ground, pulling hard on the ankles and simultaneously raising your head and chest until you are poised on your abdomen. Lift the head well up and look straight ahead of you.

At first you may find it a help to widen the space between the knees for the second part of this exercise. You may not be able to achieve elevation at first. Continue to lift as far as you can without jerking, hold this position for five seconds, relax and rest. It will help the lift if you push the knees out. Gradually you will gain elasticity. Once you have managed to raise the chest and thighs, try to reduce the space between the knees and deepen your stretch.

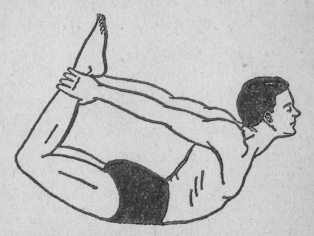

Therapeutic Value : The Bow Posture, together with the Cobra Pose which follows, are the two most important exercises for backward stretch of the spine. Meanwhile the abdominal region is stretched and exercised and the entire sympathetic nervous system stimulated. This results not only in physical well-being and longevity, but improved emotional and nervous control.

19. BHUJANGASANA, or *Cobra Pose :*
Method : Lie face down on the mat, forehead touching the ground, with arms bent so that the elbows point upward and the

palms rest on the ground just below the shoulders. Stretch the legs well out, keeping them stiff and straight, with the soles pointing upward. Do not allow the knees to slacken or bend. Now raise the head slowly, as high as possible, jutting the chin forward, feeling the stretch. Lift chest and torso off the ground, pressing down on the hands but letting the contraction of the back take most of the strain. Feel pressure traveling down the spine all the way to the sacral region. Make sure your body from the navel to the toes rests on the floor. When you are finally upright, like a cobra poised to strike, retain the pose for as long as possible without feeling undue strain. Increase the time gradually from a few seconds to a full minute. Then slowly return to the face-down position. Relax and rest.

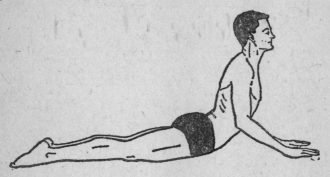

In time you will be able to dispense almost entirely with support from the hands and arms, although at first this may seem not even remotely possible. However, once perfected this *asana* gives great benefit even though it need be performed only once a day.

Therapeutic Value : An exercise to make the spine amazingly supple and flexible, at the same time it revitalizes abdominal muscles. Kidney, liver and pancreas are stimulated so that the appetite improves and bodily heat increases. This *asana* is of great value to persons who do a great deal of stooping—sedentary workers and women overburdened with housework—and all who suffer from habitual backache.

Caution : If your spine is stiff, proceed cautiously. Remember that whereas a smooth slow stretch will benefit you, a wrench may be painful or even harmful.

20. PASCHIMATANASANA, or the *Posterior Stretch*, an *asana* which brings into play muscles all over the body.

Method : Lie flat on your back, legs close together. Slowly raise the head, chest and trunk until you are sitting up, being careful never to raise the legs off the floor or bend the knees. Now exhale slowly, at the same time bending forward until you grip your toes. (If you cannot reach them, catch hold of ankles or calves; you will do better eventually.) The object of this exercise is to touch your knees with your face while keeping the legs fully extended. This stretch will create a sharp curve at the base of the spinal column. Bend as far forward as you can without jerking, hold the position for ten seconds, then slowly return to upright sitting position. Inhale. Lie back and relax.

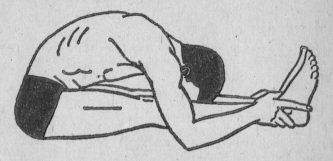

Do this exercise only once each period, being careful to maintain rhythmic motion. Maximum benefit is obtained by pulling the body a bit further each time.

Therapeutic Value : This Deep Contraction has the opposite effect of that based on Bhujangasana. The abdominal muscles are vigorously contracted and massaged; the spine is stretched the opposite way; the liver squeezed; the sex gland and the nerves at the base of the back are toned up. The posterior muscles, which are seldom properly exercised, are thoroughly stretched. Practiced in conjunction with Bhujangasana, this *asana* makes for physical rejuvenation, and also stimulates the kidneys and pancreas. It is especially recommended for women, since it envigorates the pelvic region and keeps abdominal muscles under control, melting away any surplus fat.

21. HALASANA, or the *Plough Pose :*
Method : Lie flat on your back with legs stretched out. Keeping the knees stiff, raise the legs to an angle of thirty degrees. Hold this position for five seconds, then raise the legs another thirty degrees. Again hold for five seconds. Now raise them until they

are in a vertical position, hold for two seconds, then *slowly* swing them over your head until the tips of your toes touch the floor behind your head. Be careful at all times to keep the knees stiff and the palms of your hands flat on the floor, arms straight.

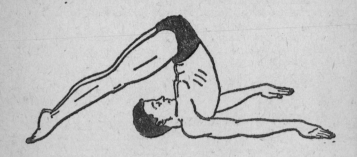

Next slide your toes further away from your head, always remembering to keep the knees stiff. Feel the weight shift toward the top of the spine until it is supported mainly by the vertebrae of the neck. Hold this final position fifteen to twenty seconds, then gradually reverse your movements until you are again flat on your back. Relax and rest.

Remember to breathe deeply and regularly throughout this exercise. You will doubtless have difficulty at first in touching the floor with your toes unless you do bend your knees. Also, the palms of your hands will tend to lift off the floor. Try to keep them down. When you have perfected this *asana*, one performance of it daily, sustained for thirty seconds, is all you will need. The aim is a single prolonged stretch, not several repetitions, although repetition is what you will inevitably get at first.

Therapeutic Value : This *asana* stretches spine and abdominal muscles, helps circulation and thyroid action, and consequently helps prevent arthritis. It also continues the beneficial effects of Savasana.

22. SIRSHASANA, or *The Headstand*, traditionally associated with Yoga and second only to the Lotus or Buddha Pose in identifying the entire subject of Hatha Yoga in the Western mind. It is not nearly as difficult to do as people imagine, may be learned

at any age and, once mastered, is wonderfully relaxing and all-inclusive. However, the student should proceed cautiously at first while learning it, since recklessness or impatience may cause injury.

Method : For best results the Headstand should be practiced and learned in four stages, although once you have mastered the technique its execution will be surprisingly smooth and relaxing.

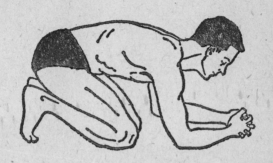

FIRST STAGE: Kneel on a mat, clasp your hands, fingers interlocked, and let both the hands and the forearms rest on the floor with elbows not too wide apart.

SECOND STAGE: Next place your head, about one inch above the forehead, within the triangle thus formed, but be sure it rests on the pad and not on the hands themselves. Cup your hands around your head so that the thumbs support it. Now slowly get up from your knees and stand on your toes. Next try to bring your toes closer in to your head, taking small steps, knees stiff. You have doubtless observed small children standing this way, bent practically in half, bottoms up. Adults do not assume this pose naturally, but you should continue to try it. Even if you never get beyond this first stage of the Headstand, you will derive benefits from it in limberness and improved circulation. However, here is a word of caution: This reverse position is not for persons with either very high or very low blood pressure, weak eye capillaries, chronic nasal catarrh or defective (not merely sluggish) pituitary or thyroid glands.

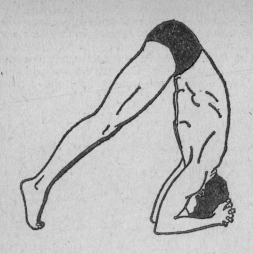

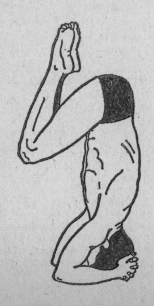

STAGE THREE: Until you are adept at the Headstand, it is wise to practice Stage Two either in a corner or against a wall, partly as insurance against falling and partly because of the sense of safety and balance you may need simply for reassurance. You may also need the help of another person at your first attempt. In that case, having assumed the first position and gotten your feet close to your head, raise one leg, then have the person helping you grasp it by the ankle and hold you while you straighten it. The other leg will follow naturally. The illustration shows the proper position, with both legs raised. If you attempt to raise your legs without help, you may find it easier to raise them both at once, giving yourself a boost as if with a slight jumping motion, knees bent.

STAGE FOUR: Then slowly raise the legs and feet and straighten them, until your entire body is vertical. The wall or corner will prevent your falling over backward. Hold this position for five seconds, then slowly lower the legs, bending the knees for balance, and finally let your feet rest on the floor once more. Get up. Lie down and relax.

The Headstand requires no special or even average strength. It will come easy as soon as you have acquired the needed sense of balance. Once you get the "feel" of this *asana* you will experience no further difficulty in performing it, but only a sense of exhilaration and relaxation. Eventually you will hold it for five minutes or more, once a day. Yogis, of course, retain this pose for thirty minutes, a whole period of meditation.

Therapeutic Value: This *asana* supplies blood to the brain, clearing the mind and helping concentration and toning the nervous system. It is recommended for developing brainpower in the young and maintaining mental health throughout life. By reversing gravity, it relieves the inevitable heart strain which accompanies normal living, thus prolonging life. The increased blood supply to the brain also improves weak eyesight, faulty hearing, sharpens all senses, cures many neurotic symptoms, improves the sense of balance and banishes insomnia. It is of great value in keeping the endocrine glands healthy, reducing all tension, fatigue and poor circulation. It is also good for the memory. In short, it is known as the "King of the Asanas," and is said to bring eternal youth. Again, however, the caution given for Stage One must be repeated: It must not be done by persons with abnormally high or low blood pressure or any of the disorders mentioned at Stage One—at least, not until they have been cured by other, simpler *asanas*.

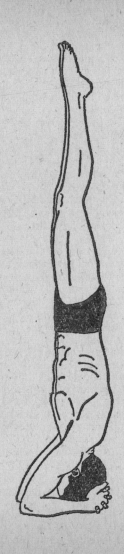

CHAPTER XII

Food and Diet:
The Healthful Yoga Way

Man is as he eateth, so George Bernard Shaw was fond of saying. He happened to be a vegetarian on principle, but whether or not he would have lived to his 94 years had his diet included meat no one can say. One thing is certain, however.

His frugal habits, his abstemiousness, his spareness of body doubtless had a great deal to do with his long life and vigorous health.

It is not *what* we eat that is of paramount importance, but *how* we eat, when and how much. Always remember that eating really includes not only the intake of food but its digestion and assimilation. In a sense, breathing should be considered part of the process too, since bodily nourishment must of necessity include the intake of oxygen; the more oxygen is inhaled into your lungs, the better fed and cleansed your blood-stream will be.

Keep in mind the fable about the senses: "Without breath there can be no life." It is possible to exist on breath alone for many days while fasting, but the most perfectly balanced diet could not sustain you longer than a few minutes were your supply of oxygen cut off. Consequently our discussion of diet cannot be considered as separate from other aspects of your way of life.

We all know how a large meal, gobbled fast, especially when one is tired or in a state of nervous tension, may and often does produce indigestion or painful gas. So does anger. The ulcers from which high-pressure executives so often suffer are the direct result of emotional strain, for when the system is not at rest the digestive juices fail to flow freely and an acid condition is set up which, literally, corrodes the sensitive mucous lining of stomach and intestines. The habit of gulping food is in itself lethal, for the gulper starves himself even as he overeats.

Here are some of the pertinent facts which you doubtless already know but are likely to disregard in practice a couple of times a day:

Chewing food slowly and thoroughly serves a double function. First of all it is good for your teeth. Unless you give them a daily workout by chewing solid foods, they will weaken and decay for want of exercise. Secondly, unless you do chew your food properly you do not give the saliva a chance to penetrate it. Saliva is, as you know, an important digestive juice. It contains ptyalin, an enzyme which transforms starches into maltose, or body sugar. Such foods as potatoes, bread, noodles, cereals, and mealy vegetables—in other words, the carbohydrates—must all be saturated with ptyalin if they are to do the body any good. This process must be accomplished before the carbohydrates leave the mouth, for once they have been swallowed, the hydrochloric acid in the stomach prevents any further digestion. That is why fast eaters seldom grow fat regardless of the quantities of good they consume. And while you may argue that nothing could be pleasanter than being able to gorge and still stay thin, in reality this is a fine way of cheating yourself; for the net result is undernourishment and a consequent lack of energy.

Finally, chewing food thoroughly also diminishes the appetite or, to put it another way, the more you chew the less you will want or need to eat, for small amounts of food will keep you well-nourished provided, of course, that your diet is a balanced one. Taking time to taste and to savor will also enhance your enjoyment of food. And this will in turn pay added dividends, for pleasure in the tasting helps a free flow of gastric juices, which helps digestion. To put it another way, be glad if a dish that is set before you makes your mouth water.

Is it necessary to adhere to strict diet rules to follow Yoga teachings? The answer depends on each person's personal goals. The highly developed Yogi is a teetotaler and a most frugal eater, but contrary to popular misconception there are no strict rules; the Yogis are neither food faddists nor even necessarily vegetarians, and their attitude toward eating is not one of asceticism. Their general approach to diet, as to all other aspects of human behavior, is one of moderation and self-discipline. They do not consider enjoyment of food synonymous with gluttony and would never advocate robbing you of the pleasures of savoring the taste, smell, texture, even the appearance of the dishes you like. Nor do they believe there is any special virtue in vegetarianism as such—if, by that, one means helping make someone into a better man or woman. But Yoga teaches that certain foods, among them milk, fruit, cereals, butter, cheese and all vegetables (preferably eaten raw) are Sattwic food-stuffs and render the blood-stream and the mind pure; while meat, fish, eggs are Rajasic and excite the passionate nature of man. From this you may readily see how a highly detached philosopher will make a choice of foods.

Possibly the reason why so many people have come to equate vegetarianism with Yoga is that Mahatma Ghandi, that most famous of Gurus, never touched meat. That was his personal choice. The fact is, too, that the Hindee in general are not great meat-eaters. India's hot climate and its low standard of living doubtless have much to do with this, besides which in a country where the cow is a sacred animal meat consumption would naturally tend to be lower than in other parts of the world. But these are only contributing factors. Here is how one Yogi teacher explained his own preference for a diet of fruit, milk, vegetables and nuts: "My tastes have grown simpler with the years," he told me in the course of discussion. "As I became more detached, my habits, my very body needs seemed to change. I never forced it—it simply happened. Today I no longer desire meat or other rich foods." But this was a man who had spent twenty years in seclusion in a monastery. He made it clear that he did not expect his disciples to follow his strict regimen.

Since Yoga principles for mental and physical health coincide so amazingly with the findings of modern medicine, it is not surprising to find their basic diet rules similar to the health diets advocated by our own up-to-date experts. The accent, as already mentioned, is on fresh fruit and vegetables, high-protein foods like eggs, cheese, meat in small quantities, nuts, and milk, modest amounts of fats and carbohydrates—and as few condiments as possible. It is important to eat natural, not processed foods, in order to get the full benefit of what the earth can give us.

There are many vitamins, minerals and other elements necessary to human diet, and if you wish to know them in detail any good book on nutrition will list them for you. In a general way, though, all you need to remember is how to cater to the body's three vital vitamin needs—how to supply it with sufficient amounts of Vitamins A, B and C and give it enough protein and mineral. A good rule to remember is that few foods are so specialized they give you one thing only. You are more than likely to get adequate amounts of everything your body requires if you make sure that its main demands are cared for through a balanced, common-sense diet.

Vitamin A is what enables the body cells to resist infection. It is contained in green and leafy vegetables, dairy products, fruit and meat, especially liver and lamb. Along with this vitamin you will be absorbing calcium, iron and the much-needed body-building proteins. And if you substitute fish for some of the meat, you will be getting precious iodine without recourse to iodized salt, which sometimes makes the skin break out.

The Vitamin B-Complex influences digestion. Whole wheat is one excellent source of this vitamin. Unfortunately, bread made with commercially-prepared flour is hopelessly impoverished. It is, in fact, almost wholly devitalized, its bran, natural minerals and semolina removed, the living wheat germ isolated and sold separately for good money while the "dead" flour must now be artificially "enriched" or "fortified," another process that adds to its cost. Thus white bread is virtually valueless nutrition-wise. Your best available sources of Vitamin B, in this day and age, are dark bread, nuts, peas, beans, lentils, cabbage and brussel sprouts, soy beans and yeast; also the dairy products and liver already listed under Vitamin A.

Digestion is not the only thing controlled by this Vitamin group. As you probably know, massive doses of the B-Complex, given by injection, have proved effective in the treatment of arthritis and that little-known degenerative disease of the nerve endings, multiple sclerosis. For regeneration of tissues and maintaining healthy nerves scientists recognize it as being of paramount importance. And more is being learned about its importance every year.

Vitamin C is the youth-preserver as well as the substance that keeps you from getting colds, and helps combat them if they settle in. The best source of this vitamin is the citrus fruit family—oranges, lemons, limes and grapefruit. These should be squeezed fresh and never strained, for the pulp is too precious to throw away. Tomatoes and tomato juice are a second good source. Lacking either, there is some Vitamin C in potato jackets and also in turnip greens and spinach. But remember, this is a volatile vitamin which does not keep, nor can it be stored in the body. Consequently, you need your daily allotment regularly.

Before we leave the subject of vitamins, it is important to point out what processing does to foods in general. Rice, for instance, like wheat, is robbed of half its nutrients while it is elegantly polished, then processed for quick cooking. The canning process, while often unavoidable, destroys much that is valuable. Then the average cook, out of habit or ignorance or because of a desire to serve food that looks pretty, robs her family by discarding the green outside leaves of lettuce and romaine, by peeling potatoes instead of either baking them or cooking them in their jackets, and by overcooking vegetables and throwing away the water—and half the vitamins and minerals with it. There is also the tendency to buy fresh vegetables in quantity and to store them in the refrigerator, allowing much of their nutritive value to be lost. In fact, we are constantly committing sins against our stomachs simply because we do not stop to think about the right way to eat.

But even before we have a chance to ruin food ourselves, and before it has been processed, part of the job is already done by the grower. Fruit and vegetables out of season, as well as jumbo-size and picture-pretty food, bring high prices. Consequently the grower forces his produce with various chemicals. And these chemical fertilizers result in food that is tasteless (in our family the word for the winter tomato, for instance, is "factory-made," and I know of no better way to describe it!), but, what is far more serious, chemicals are not an adequate source of basic nutrients. That is why so many health authorities continually stress the importance of naturally grown foods—which means foods grown in soil enriched with natural fertilizers—garden compost, manure, bone meal, wood ashes and so forth.

We cannot all have truck gardens and raise our own crops, but it helps to understand the following basic facts about nutrition and at least follow certain simple rules:

1. Fruit and vegetables are best bought in season, and only in quantities which can be utilized fairly fast.
2. Whenever possible, do not discard peelings. On the other hand it is essential to wash fruit and vegetables carefully, not only because they have been handled but because they may have a residue of some poisonous spray, such as arsenic or DDT, clinging to them. However, if produce are to be stored, do not wash until ready to serve. This is especially true of berries.
3. Both fruit and vegetables are best eaten raw, but if you must cook them, cook only until just soft, never to limpness. Bring the water to a boil first, use very little of it to begin with, and if possible, allow this to be re-absorbed. Try to utilize any remaining vegetable water in sauces or soups. An even better method is steaming.
4. In flavoring, learn to substitute herbs, garlic, lemon

juice and onion for heavy quantities of salt, pepper and spices. Monosodium glutamate (sold under the trade name Accent, but much cheaper if bought by weight in the drugstore) which is not a condiment, helps bring out the natural flavor of foods by stimulating our taste buds, which through indiscriminate use of catsup, meat sauces and other sharp flavorings have become jaded. Learn to use it, unless of course you are on a salt-free diet, in which case it will not be permitted.

5. Finally, learn to enjoy foods prepared simply, without rich sauces which only mask the natural taste and add unnecessary calories. Remember that broiled foods are better for you than fried. And never drown your food by drinking with your meals.

There are certain foods which require special mention here:

Garlic is said in some parts of the world to have magic properties. Italian peasant women will carry a head of it in their pocket or wear whole garlands of it like beads to keep epidemics away. Sanskrit writings of 2,500 years ago also mention its therapeutic values. As sometimes happens, old wives' tales and legend turn out to coincide with medical facts. Recent research bears out the claim for garlic as a curative agent in the treatment of stomach, blood and catarrhal complaints such as influenza. In fact, pure garlic oil is now available in small, soluble capsules for those who cannot bear its taste and odor. But there is more pleasure in cultivating a liking for it.

Olive oil is a fine lubricant for the system as well as a source of easily-digested vegetable fat. People who must worry about the cholesterol content of their blood are advised to substitute peanut or other vegetable oil, both of which are also preferred by some for their neutral taste. However, the calorie content of a spoonful of oil need not worry you if you follow your Yogi routine so that your food is digested properly—and if you do not overeat on such rich foods as cream sauces and rich pastries.

As a general rule, *honey* is better for sweetening than sugar. In fact, honey is one of the most easily digested of foods, for

it is transformed in a matter of minutes into blood-sugar, pro-
viding new energy and dissipating fatigue. The secret of honey
is known to most athletes. A spoonful of pure honey, swallowed
plain if you are a honey fancier, or diluted in a glass of warm
water, will stimulate you like a glass of whiskey, but without
the side effects.

Molasses—not to be confused with the commercially-sold
black treacle—is another quick source of energy and can be
assimilated by the weakest stomach. Pure molasses may generally
be obtained in health food stores. It is an especially desirable
adjunct to one's diet because it is said to prevent hair from
turning gray. Pure maple syrup is another fine source of
nourishing sweetening, as is raw sugar. Brown sugar is better
than white. And "refined" sugar is at the bottom of the list.

Because adulteration of food is actually inevitable in our
urban centers due to problems of transportation, supply and
preservation in large quantities, it is a good idea to supplement
the diet with wheat germ, soy beans and all manner of whole-
grain cereals generally considered exotic. A visit to any reput-
able health food store will give you some notion of what is
available. You will find the foods there relatively expensive,
but not as expensive in the long run as the vitamin pills so
many people depend on. Try cultivating a taste for such
"peasant" foods as black Russian pumpernickel, buckwheat
groats, the near-Eastern couz-couz which is a form of whole-
grain cereal, slow-cooking Irish oatmeal and the equally slow
brown rice. These are the staples on which millions of people
all over the world exist, and they are not undernourished
although they may be much poorer in pocket than we are.

You have already been warned against drowning food with
drink. Too many people have the habit of drinking water with
meals (or soda pop, beer or coffee), thus diluting the digestive
juices before these have had a chance to do their work. If the
food leaves the stomach only partially digested, it cannot be
properly absorbed through the walls of the intestines. Pushing
food down with liquid has yet another bad result: it makes us
eat more than we need, for after washing one portion down

we are ready for a second helping. The same is true of wine taken with a meal. Of course, a small glass taken with dinner on festive occasions does no one harm.

This brings us logically to the question everyone asks sooner or later. What is the Yoga position on alcohol in general? And again the answer, for the Western student, is moderation. There is no prohibition against liquor as such. But it would be inconceivable for a Yogi to get drunk; the advanced Yogis do not touch alcohol, since they become more and more frugal with time, preferring pure water. However, if you enjoy wine, beer and whiskey, by all means continue having them, but in small amounts.

The same may be said of tobacco. An occasional cigarette, cigar or pipe never hurt anyone. Some Hindu Yogis smoke; many Chinese ones do. Unfortunately, it is easier for the average man or woman to regulate the drinking than the smoking habit. Persons who worry about it are generally heavy smokers already and seem powerless to cut down. For them, the only answer is to cut out smoking altogether, as an alcoholic must cut out liquor, for it becomes an all-or-nothing proposition. Other people do not have the same problem. As for non-smokers, especially young people who have not yet begun using tobacco in earnest, perhaps the best answer would be not to begin at all in order to avoid all danger of becoming enslaved by habit.

Now for the drinking of liquids in general: the best drink of all, the Yogis claim, is pure cool water, of which the body requires six to eight glasses a day. Although not itself a food, water is nevertheless a life-giving substance, and the liquids within our tissues must constantly be replenished. We eliminate water constantly, largely through our sweat glands, and this is true even when we are not conscious of sweating. It is a continuous process, like breathing, necessary for the proper elimination of poisons. Water is also vital for flushing the kidneys properly, for cleansing the blood, and for proper elimination through the intestines.

The Yogi practice is to have a glass of water immediately upon rising, a final glass before going to bed at night, and several glasses in between meals. This water is never iced, but merely cool—at room temperature or even a bit warmer. Ice water and all iced drinks are one of civilization's more harmful inventions, for they impair digestion, produce stomach cramps and crack the enamel on the teeth.

Other drinks that are highly beneficial are fresh fruit and vegetable juices, which we already mentioned in our discussion of vitamins. Frozen and canned juices are not as rich in vitamins, but still valuable. It is a good general rule not to let juice stand more than a day in the refrigerator once it has been squeezed or opened, for some of the vitamins will inevitably be lost.

Milk is the only liquid which may be taken *with* a meal, for although it is nine-tenths water, it is the most complete of foods and should be treated as such. A glass of whole milk provides all the protein you need at one meal. It should be sipped slowly, alternating with a few morsels of non-protein food. Modern dieticians advise that a pint of milk be included in the diet of every adult, and double that amount in the diet of children and pregnant women; but this quantity includes milk derivatives, such as cheese and butter. For persons watching their calorie intake skim milk, buttermilk and yogurt are even better, since all of these have most of the butterfat removed. Moreover, the culture added to yogurt and buttermilk to promote fermentation is extremely beneficial for the organism, destroying bacteria and seeming to prolong life. In the Near East, where fermented milk has been used for centuries (koumiss, an equivalent of yogurt but made with mare's milk, is a favorite food with Bulgarians and Tartars) people often live to a hale and hearty eighty, ninety or even a hundred, and the claim is that fermented milk is the secret. The East European peasant does equally well on clabber, a similar food.

Before we leave the subject of liquids, a word of warning about tea, coffee and drinks like soda-pop and cola. Americans are a nation of inveterate coffee and cola drinkers, and—this may be hard on some of you—but the fact is that numberless cups of coffee, or tea, in the course of a day are a stimulant which the body is better off without; that sweet drinks are mostly sugar and water which do nothing for you except leave a residue of sugar in your mouth to attack your teeth; and that cola drinks fill your system with harmful, habit-forming narcotics. Of course, there is no need to be rigid; a cup of coffee after dinner, or tea for a mid-afternoon pickup, can do little harm. But six or eight cups in the course of a day may leave you feeling sickish, cause gas, nausea and certainly insomnia. Also, unless you like your coffee unsweetened and black, you are likely to fill your stomach with a lot more sugar and cream than you realize, accumulating empty calories and spoiling your appetite for more useful foods.

Many people are curious about the Yoga practice of fasting and want to know how this applies to ourselves. Much has been written, along rather spectacular lines, about how Yogis sometimes go without touching food for days and even weeks. This is true, but it is nothing for the Western student to experiment with. Prolonged fasting, unless one has been trained for it, can only be harmful. On the other hand, just as it is advisable to learn to eat a little less at each meal than we think we need, to leave the table always with a slight feeling of "room for a bit more," so it is good occasionally to skip eating for a day. In fact, if you can arrange it without fuss, try making a practice of giving your stomach a day's rest once every month. This automatically will help keep your appetite in check, promote healthy elimination, and will force your body to burn up whatever unneeded reserves it may be accumulating. Naturally, however, on fast-days you are free to drink all the fruit juice you want along with plenty of water. Another good plan is to go on a diet of nothing but milk one day out of the month.

Fasting, or cutting down drastically on food, is also often recommended when one is ill. But actually the decision as to whether or not to eat at such times may be left largely to your own instincts. "Feed a cold and starve a fever" is a safe generalization, but only a generalization at best. A sick animal will not touch food. Neither will you if your system warns you not to. But if you have enough appetite to feel hunger pangs, food is probably just what you need. The main thing is never to eat simply because meal-time has rolled around. Never stuff. Do not be afraid to skip an occasional meal.

All in all, a frugal, balanced diet rich in vitamins, minerals, proteins, calcium and roughage will soon begin to pay off in improved health and a sense of well-being and will have an effect on your appearance as well. You will find your weight adjusting to the optimum for you, whether you start out too fat or too thin. If you have been suffering from constipation, you will experience relief. Your muscle tone will improve, your skin and eyes will become clear and youthful and the hair will begin to take on new sheen. Naturally part of this will be due to the exercises we hope you will be doing right along. But nutrition itself invariably plays a large role as a beauty aid. Moreover, you will sleep better and feel more relaxed, for your very nerves will be better nourished.

A well, but lightly nourished, body also results in a new alertness of mind, a serenity and a positive attitude toward other people which the average Westerner rarely experiences. Around us, too many persons live to eat. The Yogi, on the contrary, eats to live—but even while he lets his mind soar above the earth, he does not allow himself to be superior or indifferent to its products, food included. *Sama*, tranquility or control of thoughts by withdrawing the mind from worldly affairs, is the final aim of Yoga. It need not be the aim of the average student. It is enough for you to remember that food is provided for your benefit, and that it is well to take an intelligent attitude toward it. Food, like friends, must be chosen with discretion.

CHAPTER XIII

Yoga and Sex

Contrary to what many people believe, the Yogis are no more ascetics in the matter of sex than of food even though some of their elder sages do live on a lofty spiritual plane where all things of the flesh have ceased to matter. On the contrary, Yoga, being a philosophy singularly free of both puritanism and hypocrisy, its disciples recognize the sex urge for the healthy instinct it is and would consider any attempt at its suppression profoundly unhealthy. Suppression and denial can lead only to physical upsets and mental harm. It is we Westerners who sometimes tend to look on sex as unclean. But the Yogis are steeped in the general Eastern attitude which is simply that sexual impulses, like any other natural urges, may be used to either good purpose or evil, depending on ourselves.

If sex is made synonymous with physical love—the carnal side of deep and genuine emotion—it becomes a supremely meaningful and beautiful expression of the man-woman relationship, the ultimate union. Debased, it debases and brings down the misuser to animal level. The Hindus believe that woman is the complementary part of man, a gift from heaven, man's soul companion and helpmate, and that union must be not only mental and spiritual, but physical. Marriage is entered upon in an attitude of humility, with full recognition of its solemnity. In fact, one of the basic Hindu writings, the *Kama Sutra*, is an elaborate treatise on the philosophy and etiquette of love, courtship and sexual behavior, both male and female, detailed in a manner which our best modern manuals on marriage techniques do not begin to approach.

Hindu temples are often decorated with phallic represen-
tations which shock the Occidental traveler, but which to the
worshippers have a deep spiritual significance. Because of this
cultural attitude Oriental women share with their men an
approach at the same time more natural and more sophisticated,
quite unlike so many Western women who consider all sex
relationships, including that with a husband, as slightly unclean
if not indecent, a grim "duty" to be performed as the price of
staying married. In this—unfortunately for ourselves and
fortunately for the rest of the world—we are truly unique.
For there is nothing unclean about sex except the mind of the
man or woman who either is obsessed with it or cannot face it.
What is perverted is the cultural aura handed down to us from
repressed Victorian ancestors whose neurotic patterns have
helped misshape some of our own.

The Yogis, who teach that man's supreme goal is Self-
realization, understand that such realization cannot be wholly
achieved except through union with woman, his other half.
What one sex lacks the other provides. Rigid denial is merely
a superficial form of escape which is self-defeating. To live
fully, with understanding, each human being must know
something of the innermost depths of the mind of the other
sex. It is impossible to advance to complete understanding of
Self, and of the world at large, while living in ignorance of the
other half of mankind. Man and woman have been created for
each other, not to exist in separate vacuums.

However, Self-realization may not be equated with self-
indulgence. Therefore Yoga teaches that much of our sex
drive must also be sublimated, that is, channeled into other life
drives, creative or otherwise useful and always constructive.
In this Yoga is not too different from the Freudian theory
which claims that all man's urges, including the life urge itself,
are based in the *libido*. The very symbol of Kundalini, remember, is the serpent; and the serpent is one of the basic and
universal symbols of male sexuality, not only in Freudian
language but throughout mythology and folklore everywhere.
Thus in Genesis, the serpent enters the Garden of Eden and

prevails upon Eve to taste of the fruit of the Tree of Life so that she might have knowledge of good and evil. This, according to some authorities, symbolizes sex and the creative power wrongly used. It has also been pointed out that a close parallel exists between the Genesis legend and the sacred Hindu writings relating to Kundalini, for that too is generally described as "the slumbering serpent." Furthermore, when this serpent is awakened and used grossly merely to satisfy sheer animal desire—when it is directed downward to the lower physical centers—it brings knowledge of evil; directed upward toward the heart and head, it brings knowledge of good.

The Yogis themselves have learned how to transmute sex energy into psychic channels. Thus it is never either actually suppressed or dissipated but rather transmuted. Sometimes it is drawn to the solar plexus for utilizing in healthful physical exercise. Sometimes it is sent to the brain and toward the spirit. To the advanced Yogi it then brings poise, harmony, freedom from desire, lasting serenity, and finally a merging with the Universal Consciousness. To us average individuals, control over this basic inner force may well mean a happier personal life.

The man and woman doesn't exist whose personal life is not closely related to his sex life, be this good, indifferent or bad. The well-adjusted, well-functioning and sexually potent individual dreams of perpetuating this state of affairs indefinitely. The ineffectual man, the frigid woman, even if they may not realize it themselves, wish helplessly for a solution to their special problems, a solution that would bring them liberation.

Yoga offers many such solutions. In the first place, a number of the Yoga exercises help sublimate a restless sex urge while others awaken a sluggish body. Restlessness becomes positive, creative energy which may then be properly utilized instead of merely bringing trouble. Conversely, lack of interest in one's mate—and sometimes the free-floating hostility arising out of such feelings—slowly gives way to a warmer, more giving attitude.

Sex, as we all know, is not all there is to a good marriage but it is one of its cornerstones. A warmhearted partner mated with a cold, unresponsive one may be willing out of loyalty to put up with a physical starvation diet, but is bound to be adversely affected and sometimes even emotionally destroyed. Or else, the marriage itself is destroyed when once the rejected partner, having had enough of indifference, turns elsewhere for affection. Contrary to what many Westerners have been brought up to believe, primness, excessive reserve, overemphasis on decorum (the so-called virtues of the "good" woman) often are not virtue at all but a mask for deep insensibility, for an inability to love and be loved, to give and to share, or even for a need to destroy the mate, castrate him physically, so to speak, as an expression of hostility to the opposite sex. The sexless male—not as rare as many imagine—is the same kind of emotionally impoverished individual.

Yoga spiritual education frees the student of the straight-jacket of prudishness and of hostility. But long before such emotional growth has been achieved certain obvious changes may be brought about through the daily performance of the proper *asanas* and *mudras*. As we have said so many times at various points in this discussion, there can be no under-estimating of the interplay of the physical and the spiritual in the human makeup. Therefore putting your physical house in order will do wonders for you in other ways too.

Sluggish sex urges are often traceable to inadequately func-tioning endocrine glands and a resulting hormone deficiency. The gonads, or sex glands, would be the offenders here. But the gonads, like the other endocrines, are themselves controlled by the pituitary gland which is known to secrete about a dozen hormones that stimulate the proper functioning of all the other seven pairs. It may very well be, therefore, that the sexually indifferent person's basic trouble lies in some malfunctioning of the pituitary, a condition which Western medicine would treat by means of expensive hormone injections or equally expensive pills. The Yoga method, of course, is through exercise.

Turn back to the chapter on basic *asanas*, Chapter XI.

You will find that the Headstand, or *Sirshasana* (Pages 136–

139), if practiced regularly, will stimulate the pituitary gland by
sending a vast flow of blood to the head as your body briefly
defies the laws of gravity. Thus stimulated, it will then immediately wake up the gonads, which will begin to respond by
producing hormones of their own. Needless to say this is not
the only beneficial result of the Headstand (its various therapeutic effects are detailed along with directions for executing
it) but it happens to be the effect which concerns us here.

For persons unable to do the Headstand, there is the Shoulder
Stand, or *Sarvangasana* (Page 125) and the Reverse Posture,
or *Viparitakarani Mudra* (Pages 119–121), both of which
accomplish almost, if not quite, the same results. Again, you
will find a careful description of these exercises and the various
benefits derived from them in Chapter XI.

But revitalizing the pituitary is not the only way to keep the
gonads in top functioning condition. Exercises for both stimulating and sublimating the sex instincts include the Stomach Lift
or *Uddiyana Bandha* (Page 129), the Plough or *Halasana* (Pages
135–136), the Fish Pose, *Matsyasana* (Pages 123–124) and the
Supine Pelvic Posture (Page 124). Keep in mind that each of
these *asanas* is beneficial in more ways than this one—that by
learning to do them you will be reaping fringe benefits, but
their specific value here is revitalization of the gonad secretions,
overcoming seminal weakness in men and ovarian disturbances
in women. The Stomach Lift, for instance, massages the inner
walls of the abdomen and tones all stomach muscles. The
Plough, Fish and Supine Poses strengthen and stimulate the
muscles and organs of the lower abdomen, or the entire pelvic
region. This, of course, has a direct bearing on the glands
situated there. At the same time all of these *asanas* as well as the
Headstand have a beneficial effect on the thyroid gland so
closely related to our overall physical well-being.

Naturally, as has been said elsewhere, it is not necessary to
perform all of the exercises mentioned here. You would probably not have time for them even if you have the agility. Besides, in working out a schedule for yourself you must not
neglect other aspects of your Yoga routine. Since any one of

them, done accurately and regularly, will accomplish the desired results, start with whichever is easiest for you and suits you best. Keep to it for a while and, if you have time for more or wish to vary your routine, experiment with a second or a third later on. In a short while the effects will become apparent and will doubtless surprise you: you will be rewarded not only by physical revitalization, but a sense of greater inner harmony. Anxieties relating to your sexual activity will gradually vanish. This combination of renewed vitality and inner peace will eventually mean the ability to maintain undiminished sexual powers for decades longer than is generally common in the West.

Sexual potency and responsiveness—or conversely the ability to control too-violent, disturbing urges—will not be the only gain you will notice. Your instinctive drives once properly channeled, you will discover that your general relationships with others are gradually changing for the better. First and foremost, of course, there may be a change in the relationship with husband or wife. Physically and emotionally you will find yourself growing more giving, and inevitably you will receive more in turn. What's more, your new inner balance will make it possible for you to have a deeper understanding of your partner, a new responsiveness to the other's needs, a greater tolerance of faults and imperfections. What was once a simple physical urge will have grown into spiritual experience.

Aristophanes, in Plato's *Symposium*, tells how once upon a time all human beings were born like Siamese twins. Each had two heads, two sets of arms and legs and, because each was completely within the self, infinite ability and strength. So powerful did the human race grow that the gods became frightened. So to lessen the threat to themselves they severed each human creature in half. Then they scattered the halves, hopelessly mixed up, far and wide over the earth. And ever since then, each of us must spend his life groping, searching for the lost other half. A few, a very few, succeed. When this happens there is a perfect, an ideal marriage. But more often people merely *think* they have found their destined mate. Betrayed by primitive longing, they settle for a pedestrian partnership with someone whose temperament is quite incompatible with their own, then both spend the rest of a lifetime in a state of armed neutrality. Then, until death do them part the disenchanted partners bicker, undermine and hurt one another. How much more constructive to learn to search for what may be good and worthwhile in an admittedly imperfect relationship. This is what the pursuit of Yoga enables the student to do.

Learning how to sublimate the sex urge is, then, a way to develop spiritual strength. Directing the emotions toward goals of universal love means reaching out toward everything in this world that is alive and good. Thus many consider Christ a perfect example of the Yoga ideal, for His was an all-embracing love that enveloped all humanity. It was this love that made it possible for Him to say of Mary Magdalen, "Her sins, which are many, are forgiven for she has loved much . . ." Love like this of course transcends the limits of sexual emotion and those who are able to experience it come to know an inner happiness denied less understanding and compassionate natures.

In their all-embracing approach the Yogis strive to achieve purification of spirit through four stages: *Maitri*, or friendliness toward those who are contentedly happy; *Maruna*, or compassion for those who are not; *Mudita*, or gladness toward those who are virtuous; and *Upeksha*, or indifference with regard to the wicked, or rather indifference to wickedness, which nevertheless does not exclude good will and a hope that the erring may be regenerated. Along with this, there is a complete exclusion of the emotion of hate.

The very last thing a Yogi would maintain is that one must rise *above* sex. On the contrary, Yoga teaches that it is desirable to rise *by means of it* to greater spiritual heights. Properly used, sex is the greatest of gifts and none may despise its rich potentialities. Both sexes should therefore learn to accept themselves completely, man as man, woman as woman, while at the same time recognizing that each of us carries some of the qualities of the opposite sex within us. Armed with this knowledge and understanding, using sex as an adornment, it is then possible to glory in its possession, not stifle it.

CHAPTER XIV

Yoga and a Long Life

To quote George Bernard Shaw a second time, youth is wasted on the young. Of course, like all paradoxes this one can be shot full of holes, for who would really grudge young people their vitality and their joy of living! Yet it is also true that the young seldom fully savor the gifts with which the gods so liberally endow them. Some things they take too much for granted, others they cannot enjoy to the hilt because their emotions and mental capacities have not yet developed in depth.

Later on, after we have grown and learned, many of us wish for a second chance at youth, knowing we would live it more fully, find values we once never dreamed were there for the taking, develop potentials within ourselves we once let go to waste. If only we had it to do over again, we sigh nostalgically.

But it wouldn't work, if you stop to think about it. To get the most out of such a second chance we should have to be both young and old at once, wise before our time and perceptive as no untutored young mind—save possibly a genius— ever can be. And yet a second chance *is possible* through Yoga. The clock will not be turned back, nor would we really want it to be. Instead, at a time when our emotions have matured, our tastes fully formed and our wisdom (we hope) ripened, we may experience a kind of second youth by preventing the slowing-down and deterioration processes, and lengthening the span of our productive years.

A long life is not of itself necessarily a boon. Certainly it wouldn't be desirable if we were merely going to drag on, vegetating like withered apples, helpless and listless and full of infirmities, useless to ourselves and to others. But the old man or woman who retains a zest for living and knows how to relish each day's experiences, one who instead of mourning lost opportunities accepts the advantages of the present, is a rich and fortunate human being. Especially fortunate is the one who to the very end remains hale, vigorous, free of illness and pain and fears, and whose philosophy endows him with the serenity and dignity becoming to his years.

Nor is a serene old age our only goal. First there are the middle years which can and should be productive and satisfying. Earlier in the book we discussed the restlessness and tensions which beset most of us Westerners, poisoning the emotional climate in which we live. But we have still another lurking enemy to cope with: from early middle age on, sometimes even from early adulthood, we allow ourselves to become obsessed with the *fear* of growing old.

In this country especially, the cult of youth, perpetuated through the motion picture and TV screen, the advertising media, the glamor business, is so strong that men and women alike develop phobias about the onset of age. They watch anxiously for the first gray hair, the first tell-tale wrinkle, considering themselves has-beens the moment the bloom of first youth is gone. They actually speed deterioration by becoming resigned to it. Men in their thirties accept potbellies, women sagging bodies after childbirth. From there it is only one logical step to defeat via such degenerative diseases as arthritis, heart ailments and arteriosclerosis, and all because of the fatalistic assumption that whatever is wrong just has to be. Most depressing of all is the added conviction that sexual potency must inevitably diminish and desire wane as women approach the menopause and men the climacteric. In fact a good many people positively invite old age through their attitudes.

None of this is really in the cards.

Man—and woman too of course—is only as old as his endocrine glands. Keep these in top order and the advancing years need not be a menace. Your arteries, your joints, your circulatory system will continue to serve you well. This doesn't mean you will not grow old at all. Of course you will! But the aging process will proceed a great deal more slowly than you believe it possible and as a result you will feel no reluctance at progressing from one stage of life to the next, for you will be entirely ready for it.

Each age has its own appeal and also its drawbacks. Each is an experience you would not want to miss. Thus childhood and youth have special charms, but their grace is counter-balanced by inexperience and emotional turmoil. As we grow older we acquire understanding, tolerance, appreciation and self-confidence. We also become more self-sufficient, gain in judgment, financial stability and greater freedom of action and of choice. On the other hand we carry a heavier load of re-sponsibility. Others begin to expect more of us. It is no longer enough to be as the lilies of the field.

If you were granted your wish by a fairy godmother, would you really choose always to remain eighteen? Of course not. The very idea would bore you. People who are honest with themselves often say they wouldn't go through their youth again for anything in the world. Once was enough! The grow-ing pains had been just too painful. But if the good fairy offered you the boon of always functioning at the peak of your potential, that would be something else again. To thinking people, that is the only kind of eternal youth worth bothering about. And that is what Yoga offers.

If you traveled in India, you would quickly see that the Yogis in general have found the secret of the magic fountain. Not only do they live much longer than ordinary people—but they age differently. Over the decades their skins retain a smooth unlined look and their hair remains black. Their eyes are clear and their bodies supple. At eighty they look forty, for neither their minds nor their physique show impairment. Still later they may grow thin to the point of emaciation, but mentally they retain their full powers until they are ready to depart this life.

By now you can appreciate how much of this is due to the Yogi's philosophical and spiritual orientation and also to his ability to relax at will. Through relaxation he can attain the lengthening of his life span exactly as animals do—something we discussed in detail in Chapter VI. He doesn't wear himself down, he contributes nothing in self-destruction. Regular periods of meditation, on the other hand, have taught him a detachment, a preoccupation with spiritual matters on the highest level, an indifference to his surroundings, which bring inner peace and are like a shield against the encroachments of the physical world.

He has also learned over the years how to move, stand, sit, even lie down in a way to conserve every ounce of energy possible. He has conquered hate, rancor, petty annoyance and irritation. The whole arsenal of destructive emotions have long ceased to threaten him. Instead, he feels good will and love for his fellow-creatures, and these positive forces work for him.

In addition to this training of the spiritual self, the Yogi has the benefit of years of *asanas*, which he does every day. Here you have the prime and simple physical answer. Here is where all of us who would benefit from Yoga wisdom must begin. In fact, it is to be hoped that you've begun some time back—that as you have progressed through this book you have got into the habit of doing your Deep Relaxation and Dynamic Breathing exercises and that you take time for a period of Meditation each day in the *asana* or *mudra* of your choice.

In one of the earlier chapters we briefly discussed the over-all functioning of the endocrines and their bearing upon the various body processes. Since it is they that make us who we are and what we are, it is imperative to understand the role of each gland in order to safeguard their long-lasting working order. Armed with this knowledge, you will be able to orient yourself better in choosing exactly the *asanas* you need to keep yourself healthy and young.

The *pituitary* gland, at the base of the brain, secretes a number of hormones, some of which regulate body functions directly, while others affect the proper behavior of the other ductless glands. It is therefore generally considered the master gland of the body. It keeps you from becoming lazy, fat and sluggish. It regulates sugar utilization, the production of milk and the utilization of sugar, and an underactive pituitary results in diabetes. It also controls the inner mobility of the system and sexual development. Indirectly it controls our sexual behavior, largely through the influence it has on the gonads (see Chapter XIII on Sex). It is also largely responsible for our emotional well-being, and pituitary disturbance may even lead to personality changes.

The *pineal* gland, in the middle of the skull, is the body organizer or, if you will, its harmonizer. Pineal disturbance in children may cause premature development of the sex glands and of the entire system. In many ways the pineal keeps an inner balance between the other endocrine glands after the pituitary has stimulated them into functioning. In the East it is considered the seat of the sixth sense.

The *thyroid*, at the base of the neck, produces the hormone called thyroxine which increases the oxidation of the body above basal level. The thyroid is responsible for our basal metabolism rate. Thyroxine deficiency will make a person sluggish and fat, and if the deficiency is serious enough will result in cretinism, one of the most serious forms of mental deficiencies. An overactive thyroid, on the other hand, will make you thin, jumpy, nervous and tense and will increase your pulse rate. Temporary thyroid imbalances are common among women as they approach and go into menopause: sometimes this accounts for their becoming puffy (the body may not be eliminating sufficient water), for loss of hair, and dull listlessness. These symptoms are believed to be due to emotional disturbances associated with change of life, and are generally treated with gland extracts. The rate of activity of the thyroid is what makes the difference between your being alert or dull, quick or slow, vivacious or apathetic, listless or mentally keen.

The *parathyroid*, neighbor to the thyroid, controls the distribution of calcium and phosphorus in the system, which means the physical health of the nerves and of the bones. There can be no metabolic equilibrium without this gland; but its normal functioning insures poise and tranquility.

The *thymus,* which controls growth, is especially important in childhood and adolescence, since its secretions determine the proper development of the skeleton and the entire body structure. The seven-foot circus giant and the midget are both victims of thymus malfunction, which is sometimes a hereditary factor. Normally the thymus diminishes in size and importance as we reach puberty.

The *Isles of Langerhans!* in the pancreas, are the source of the hormone known as insulin, without which we do not utilize sugar properly; their improper functioning results in diabetes. Again, this lack may sometimes be brought about by severe mental and emotional strain, including the fears and despondency of change of life.

The *adrenal* glands, directly above the kidneys, control the proper flow, oxygenation and life-giving properties of blood. Properly stimulated, they supply us with adrenalin, which can drive us to action, give us courage, sharpen our perception, keep us going on "sheer nerves" when necessary. Over-stimulated, as under the stress of fear, anger or some other violent emotion, these glands will pump adrenalin into our system and cause distressing manifestations. The heart suddenly pumping too fast, the sweat, the nausea caused by anxiety are all the result of adrenalin improperly directed. In a sense the adrenals are our most primitive glands. They have never learned that civilized man cannot rid himself of emotional reaction by going into simple physical action. They continue preparing us for battle, for roaring fury or flight when convention requires us to stand still, speak softly and duel exclusively with words. They make us pay dearly for any self-confidence that is only superficial. You cannot fool the adrenal glands, but you can make good friends with them through Yoga.

The last pair of endocrines are the *gonads*—the ovaries in woman, the testes in man. Since we have already discussed them in detail in the chapter on sex, we needn't repeat. However, it must be added that their functioning is not purely a sexual one. The gonads have an effect on the whole personality. Sparkling eyes, a smooth, luminous skin, the warmth which some individuals emanate that makes them universally attractive, these are all determined by the sex glands. Conversely, the inflexibility of prematurely aging persons, the inability to establish rapport with other human beings that characterizes cold, sexless individuals and narcissistic ones, sometimes also homosexuality, are the direct results of sex hormone disturbances and deficiencies. Yet they may have nothing whatever to do with sexuality in the accepted sense.

Now that you understand the division of labor of the various glands in your body, you can readily see how important it is to safeguard their health and efficiency. Yoga exercises, beginning with deep breathing and relaxation and going on to correct stimulation of the various glandular areas, may be called the cornerstone of a program for long life and health.

Now go back to Chapter XI and read over the lists of therapeutic benefits derived from the twenty-odd *asanas* described there. You will find that some stress circulation, some strengthen the back or pelvic region, some are recommended to overcome respiratory difficulties or sluggish digestion and elimination, and still others simply benefit one òr another set of ductless glands. Depending on the time you can devote to your Yoga practice and also the condition of your body when you begin, work out a routine which will include some exercise for every organ and set of glands. Begin with the simplest and easiest; do not strain or tire yourself unduly; but make certain that your whole body is being systematically toned up. In this way you will be doing preventive therapy rather than waiting for signs of trouble which must then be cured.

If you could only do a single *asana* a day, the Headstand, provided you can master it, is doubtless the most valuable for keeping your whole system in shape. Next would be the Shoulder Stand and the Reverse Pose, done in conjunction with deep breathing. Their benefits, as you now know, are derived from the way the flow of blood to the head feeds and stimulates the pituitary which in turn stimulates the other glands. No amount of life insurance can offer you the insurance against deterioration and old age these *asanas* will provide. Their regular practice will endow you with the look of youth and the feel of youth without your ever again having to "run after" youth in undignified and unbecoming fashion.

To keep your spine straight and limber and promote good elimination, try the Camel Pose, and later the Spine and Fish Poses. You will notice that these also keep the pelvic region young and strong. The Cobra Pose combined with the Posterior Stretch makes for rejuvenation of the entire body, stimulating most of the vital organs. The Plough Posture is insurance against arthritis. Whichever *asanas* you choose, remember that in order to benefit from the very start, it is wise to work out a program that is realistic for you and relatively easy to execute. You are not trying to win prizes for achievement, or even for effort. All you want is results. Later on, as you continue to practice you will become more adventurous and start experimenting with more difficult *asanas*. By then your body will have become much more responsive and you will never want to go back to your old habits of inactivity. But do not try to rush results. And remember never to neglect relaxation poses; the Savasana and either the Lotus Pose or the Simple Pose are a must for you along with the more arduous exercises.

There is one final ingredient which *asanas* alone will never supply. Done merely as exercises, no matter how accurately and faithfully, they would remain a glorified "daily dozen" unless your mind and your spirit were fully involved. The will to change, to grow instead of ossifying, to give of yourself and to make yourself wide-open to new experiences—these too are part of the secret of eternal youth. So also is the will to live. Just as doctors agree that such a will is often the single precious factor making the difference between saving a patient and losing him, so also we cannot get along without it in our day-by-day existence. Think young and you will remain young. Think old and your joints will creak in answer.

How else can you influence your own longevity? This entire

book is really an answer to that question. If you have followed it carefully, you know by now the secrets of the trinity of mind, body and spirit which can make you over into a powerhouse of creative vitality. You know how mind influences matter while matter, in this case your nerves and muscles and blood vessels and secretions, influences mind. You know what happens when these forces work harmoniously and also the consequences of their being divided against each other.

There are a few simple rules which the Yogis follow and which might be mentioned here: Freedom being the recognition of necessity, it is wise to recognize that as we grow older we must husband our resources. We can no longer drive ourselves like youngsters and will do well to avoid fatigue and any unnecessary expenditure of energy. We need rest and sleep. On the other hand cutting down on food is advisable after the age of thirty-five. Leanness and longevity go together, as the Yogis have known for centuries and as our nutrition experts now frequently remind us.

Since it is generally agreed that senility is due to thyroid degeneration, inasmuch as in old age the thyroid normally shrinks bringing about retrogressive changes in the epithelial cells, you already know how you may avoid this process. For the rest, treat old age as a challenge. Resist it by resisting monotony, which first stultifies and finally destroys.

Very shortly after you begin your daily practice of Yoga you will find changes taking place in all your attitudes. First you will experience the physical differences: that habitual feeling of fatigue so common among us high-tension Western people will vanish. So will a score of nameless fears that bear the psychoanalytical label of anxieties. Your adrenals will no longer work overtime to tear your body apart with conflicting subsurface primitive impulses that have nowhere to go. You will see the world, and yourself in relation to it, in proper perspective.

Next your sense of values will change and you will no longer be willing to knock yourself out for unimportant rewards—no longer will you be trading your birthright for a mess of pottage. So your mind and your body, no longer at loggerheads, will stop that senseless war of attrition which can only end in the stalemate of destruction—an early grave. It takes a lifetime to learn the true art of living. But having learned it, you will give yourself a chance to enjoy the lasting fruits of this long and complex process.

CHAPTER XV

The Gift Yoga Offers You

In our modern world a long life is what most men and women are going to have. Therefore, more than at any previous time in history, how to remain healthy, active and content over the long decades is the burning problem facing countless millions. No one welcomes ripe old age if it is to be a burden. We do not want it if it is going to mean retirement and that enforced idleness which cripples the soul long before it eventually murders the body.

By devoting a mere twenty minutes or a half hour a day to the pursuit of Yoga you can, as you know by now, avoid such misery. You can enrich your life by developing your inner resources in depth, as you never before dreamed possible. You can discover within yourself inner strengths you did not suspect were there, potentials you never stopped to cultivate. In short, through Yoga you can find a new understanding of your true self and be something more than you ever were before.

Let us review first the modest minimum physical routines which will make possible your program of retraining.

First, remember to follow certain simple rules of hygiene:

Sleep enough but not too much, in a well-ventilated room but avoiding drafts, making sure that your bed doesn't sag and that you aren't smothered with too many covers. Always sleep with your head to the North and your feet to the South. In this way your body gets the benefit of the earth's magnetic currents flowing harmoniously through it in the proper direction. Your sleep will be infinitely more beneficial if you remember to do this.

In the morning try if possible to set aside a regular period for your Yoga breathing, relaxation and concentration routines, preferably combined with a few *asanas*. If you must leave these routines for later in the day, at least make sure of a few minutes given over to deep breathing before you dress. Do the breathing after you have washed, brushed your teeth and cleaned your tongue and also emptied your bladder. Try to establish the habit of evacuating your bowels at this time, too, especially if you plan on the full Yoga routine; but do not force yourself or allow the bowel movement to become a matter of concern.

After your breathing and relaxation exercises, make sure you eat breakfast without gulping. Never skip this first meal, but keep it light. It is a good general rule not to overeat: always get up from the table slightly unsatisfied, as if you could stand another mouthful.

If morning is not a good time for your Yoga exercises, be sure to allocate a regular period for them either at the end of your working day or before going to bed. But do not delay until you stagger with fatigue. If you do, it will be too late for the exercises to do you the maximum good. Do not wait until you are overtired.

Make it a practice sometime during your waking hours to take out five to fifteen minutes for complete relaxation, with your mind a blank and your body completely limp.

Remember to practice Dynamic Breathing at odd moments, whether while taking a walk or sitting relaxed in a chair.

So much for the needs of your body. As for rules of conduct, a Yogi, remember, expects to live by high standards. He must overcome fear, be honest with himself, be sincere, aware of others and must never hurt anyone. Self-knowledge is a most important goal. One of the objects of Meditation is to learn to see yourself as you really are, which isn't necessarily as others see you. Once you have reached this stage of understanding of self you will also have reached a far greater understanding of your fellow human beings. You will then experience a great sense of belonging, of oneness with those around you—something which in this age of isolation and alienation is the greatest possible boon.

Jealousy, anger, envy, hate are not only to be avoided—they

are emotions unworthy of one whose philosophy attempts to encompass true understanding of others. As your own self-searching bears fruit, you will find these unwelcome emotions more and more foreign to you. For, knowing that the shortcomings of others are no worse than your own, you will look upon them with tolerance. And as you yourself tend more and more to be well-disposed toward those with whom you come in contact, they in turn will respond with greater good will and positiveness toward you.

Tolerance, charity, compassion are to be cultivated and soon will become a happy habit. This in turn will bring its own dividends. You will find yourself more and more at peace with the world, no longer permitting the imperfections of others to act as irritants. But of course this is not your prime aim in making yourself over. Few benefits are ever reaped from good will that is forced or faked in opportunistic fashion. In your relations with others as well as with yourself always remember you must be honest. Only then can you expect to know the joy of true serenity and be able to benefit from it. For there is no pretending with the inner man!

We hope that you have been practicing Concentration and Meditation—practicing them mechanically at first if need be —and that by now they have become sufficiently a habit to carry you a step further. Where at first the object of your concentration may have been a candle-flame and your meditation centered on the petals of a flower, now you should be ready to apply the same techniques to the solution of real problems. If you have a decision to make, consider the aspects of the situation at hand from all sides, weighing the pros and cons, projecting yourself into the future, trying to visualize how you would function under the circumstances that are being created. Do not day-dream—really *concentrate* on what troubles you— and the correct answers will come to you. For the answer to every question that concerns you deeply is within yourself, and you will discover what you must do if only you let the parts of the puzzle fall in place to form a whole. Use the tools of Concentration and Meditation for this.

Sometimes you may find that, having considered every angle carefully, you want to delay your decision—sleep on it. This is an excellent approach. Not surprisingly you will discover the following morning that you know "instinctively" what you really want to do. This is the result of having permitted yourself to benefit by the subconscious functioning of association—which we sometimes call intuition at work—with your subliminal mind free to arrive at inevitable conclusions, or at least conclusions that are inevitable *for you*.

Concentration of this kind is a sure guide to future action, for it helps you act on the basis of your best and deepest instincts combined with inner knowledge, rather than on shallow impulse or because you are allowing yourself to be pushed into a decision; pushed either by others or by your own uncertain sense of values. Such concentration helps develop independence of mind and also self-sufficiency, the lack of which is nothing more nor less than a lack of faith in your own self. Learn, therefore, to think straight so that you can trust yourself fully.

Remember Pantajali's definition of Yoga as "the achievement of absolute mastery over the mind and emotions." Once a person has become fully aware of Self, this great teacher always stressed, he never again becomes so lost in what is happening in the world around him that he forgets to live a real inner life of his own.

But you must learn to live your inner life without undue tension. Introspection can mean enlightenment; it can also mean self-destruction. In the process of learning who you are and what you are, there will be a time when, having observed yourself, you will not like what you see, for deep down each of us is his own severest critic. Do not make a career of tearing yourself down. By all means analyze your present shortcomings and defects, bring them into the open plane of your mind, but do not dwell on them. Determine to change what you dislike, and start on the problem systematically, a little each day.

Try also to get a clear insight into the fears and anxieties you have been harboring. Make an actual list of them if you find that otherwise you shy away from grappling with them. Once you have done this, once you have confronted your private ghosts, you will be able to exorcise them in the clear light of day. Let the clean wind and the sunshine of lucid knowledge blow through the hidden corridors of your subconscious. You will become a new person. For, the moment you face fears, most of them turn into nothing—few are realities. It is as President Roosevelt once said, we have nothing to fear but fear itself.

The fears that are real must be faced; that which you cannot change must be accepted. But instead of letting yourself be routed you must learn to live with reality. This is not easy and cannot be accomplished in one swoop, but neither is it as hard as you may think. The main thing here is your own determination. The clear light of reason is your best ally—that is why clear thinking, achieved through Meditation and Concentration, is all-important to your new orientation. With it will come a courage you hardly suspect you possess!

It is important always to bear in mind the following three maxims:

First, a negative attitude not only presupposes failure but actually invites it. Conversely, you can think yourself into an attitude of success. This is not auto-suggestion. Your thoughts invariably determine your own actions and other people's reactions to you.

Hence the second rule—learn to act as if failure were impossible. This doesn't mean you are to become arrogant. Far from it. Self-confidence does not preclude modesty. A completely confident person, quietly aware of inner strength and ability, is more likely to be modest about it than the man or woman who must bluster because of inner insecurity. All that you must ask of yourself, then, is to maintain a completely positive attitude and to act on the positive, constructive impulses instead of on the self-defeating ones.

Thirdly, and lastly, never permit yourself to doubt that you have within you the strength and ability to overcome whatever difficulties are in your path. Simply learn—and here again Yoga Concentration is your ally—to dig out what is best in yourself and to utilize it. You are never as weak nor other people as strong as, in your moments of despondency, you may imagine. Remember to *direct* your energy and brainpower instead of allowing them to react automatically, and you will find that you have harnessed a powerhouse.

Most people allow themselves to be defeated by putting off what they want to accomplish, meaning to get things done but never doing them. Learn to see the continuity of action and events. The future is not something beyond you, but a continuation of the present, just as the present is a continuation of the past. Therefore the future will never be automatically "different" and tomorrow will not be magically "better" unless you consciously work at changing your patterns. Anything else is a vain and superstitious hope, and the sooner you recognize this the further along you will be. Success is rarely a matter of luck. More often it is a matter of marshaling your forces. Oddly enough it is not intelligence which is the decisive factor here, but determination. Highly intelligent people are often the sensitive ones who vacillate; they also allow themselves to be distracted by extraneous interests from the main tasks they have set themselves. Later on they wonder bitterly why someone less bright, and far less talented, has got ahead of them.

From this it does not necessarily follow that in order to be a success one must have a one-track mind. Rather, it is attacking one problem at a time that will make the difference. Allow yourself all the broad interests you feel you need in order to make your life rich in varied experience. But know *when* to indulge your preferences. Learn to husband your time and your energy.

The Yogis taught that there was nothing beyond human reach for him who believed he could do what he set out to do and kept on trying with complete concentration. This is an excellent thing to keep in mind. You can readily see now why concentration exercises are so very important. Having once mastered the approach, it is up to you to select your attitudes and each day perform some exercise in Dynamic Concentration.

Begin simply. Give yourself some task well within your ability and see to it that you do what you have promised yourself at the time you have set for it. Do not let interruptions distract you nor pleasure interfere. The discipline is well worth the effort. Soon you will be experiencing a real sense of delight in accomplishing necessary things which once you were forever putting off until some never-never hour. At the same time the feeling of guilt, of pressure, which procrastination generates will magically leave you.

Getting back briefly to the physical exercises, you might easily apply the concentration discipline to getting your *asanas* done. This is the best way we know of to conquer that ever-present desire to begin "tomorrow." Tomorrow never comes unless you prepare for it today; learn not to put yourself off with excuses.

As your physical well-being improves through the Yoga routines and your mind quiets down and stops playing tricks on you, you can begin to re-read this book, repeating the lessons already learned, but exploring more in depth. Always keep in mind that there is no end to learning and growth in general and that this is especially true of Yoga. Keep with it, make it a perpetual program, and you will have found the power to renew yourself, to maintain at maximum level your mental, physical and spiritual development. To many throughout the world Yoga is a gift from the gods. You can make this gift your own, for it is offered to you free if you just make a little effort. Not only will your span of life on earth have then been lengthened, but your existence will become that much happier, healthier and more harmonious.

INDEX

Mayflower Handbooks for your information